EASY EXERCISES

for

Flexibility

The Stay Fit Series

A Special Report published
by the editors of *Healthy Years*
in cooperation with UCLA Health

Easy Exercises for Flexibility: The Stay Fit Series

Consulting Editor: Ellen G. Wilson, PT, MS, Director, UCLA Therapy Services

Author: Jim Brown, PhD
Editor, Belvoir Media Group: Cindy Foley
Creative Director, Belvoir Media Group: Judi Crouse
Production: Mary Francis McGavic

Publisher, Belvoir Media Group: Timothy H. Cole
Executive Editor, Book Division, Belvoir Media Group: Lynn Russo

Print ISBN 978-1-879620-28-5
Digital ISBN 978-1-941937-79-2

To order additional copies of this report or for customer-service questions, please call 877-300-0253 or write: Health Special Reports, 535 Connecticut Avenue, Norwalk, CT 06854-1713. To subscribe to the monthly newsletter *Healthy Years*, call 866-343-1812 or write to the address above.

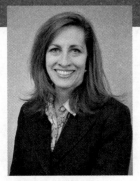

Ellen G. Wilson, PT, MS, Director, UCLA Therapy Services

*E*asy Exercises for Flexibility is part of UCLA's *Stay Fit Series*, and it may be the one that could have the quickest impact on your daily life.

The report's most important message: Don't take flexibility for granted. It is a critical component of total fitness, but one that often gets overlooked.

Although all us gradually lose flexibility as we age, new studies show that much of the loss is due to inactivity, not aging itself. You *can* do something to maintain and even improve your flexibility, and *Easy Exercises for Flexibility* can help you choose a program that fits your specific needs. If you prefer, you can design your own workouts.

To help improve your flexibility, this Special Report:

- Provides current, evidence-based information and research on fitness and flexibility (including 13 research studies)
- Helps you make informed decisions about exercise
- Offers 64 stretching and range-of-motion exercises from which to choose
- Matches exercises with your lifestyle, fitness level, and goals
- Includes tools to plan a program and record your progress

As with all the other Special Reports—*10 Activities, Aerobic Fitness, Balance & Mobility, Bones & Joints, Core Fitness, More Strength & Power, Strength & Power,* and *Walking*—*Easy Exercises for Flexibility* offers sample exercise programs and a comprehensive workbook to help you get organized, get going, and stay motivated.

Most of all, those of us at UCLA Health encourage you to stay fit and flexible for a lifetime, beginning today.

Sincerely,

Ellen G. Wilson

Ellen Wilson

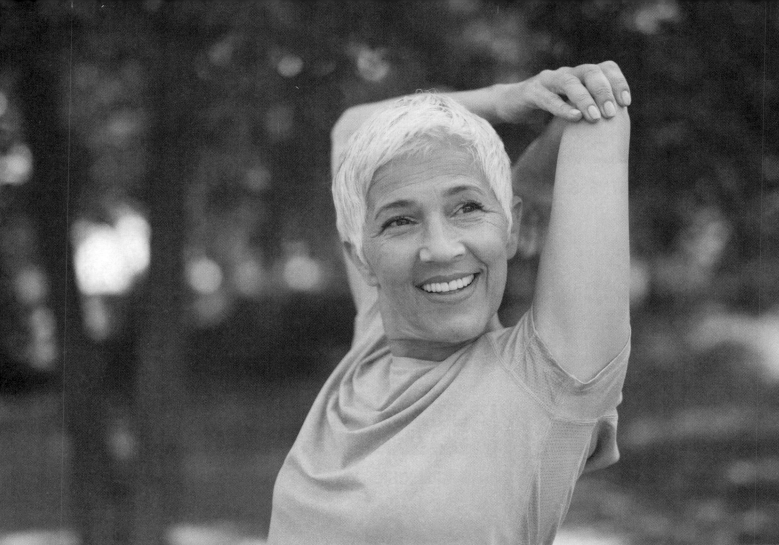

© Boggy | Dreamstime

Research Findings

1

EASY EXERCISES
FOR
AEROBIC FITNESS

THE STAY FIT SERIES

A Special Report published by the editors of HEALTHY *Years* in conjunction with

UCLA Health

2

EASY EXERCISES
FOR
BALANCE & MOBILITY

THE STAY FIT SERIES

A Special Report published by the editors of HEALTHY *Years* in conjunction with

UCLA Health

3

EASY EXERCISES
FOR
BONES & JOINTS

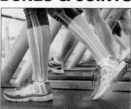

THE STAY FIT SERIES

A Special Report published by the editors of HEALTHY *Years* in conjunction with

UCLA Health

4

EASY EXERCISES
FOR
CORE FITNESS

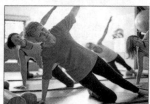

THE STAY FIT SERIES

A Special Report published by the editors of HEALTHY *Years* in conjunction with

UCLA Health

5

EASY EXERCISES
FOR
FLEXIBILITY

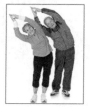

THE STAY FIT SERIES

A Special Report published by the editors of HEALTHY *Years* in conjunction with

UCLA Health

6

EASY EXERCISES
FOR
STRENGTH & POWER

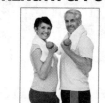

THE STAY FIT SERIES

A Special Report published by the editors of HEALTHY *Years* in conjunction with

UCLA Health

7

EASY EXERCISES
FOR
MORE STRENGTH & POWER

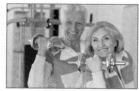

THE STAY FIT SERIES

A Special Report published by the editors of HEALTHY *Years* in conjunction with

UCLA Health

8

EASY EXERCISES
10 ACTIVITIES FOR
FITNESS & FUN

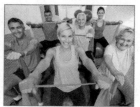

THE STAY FIT SERIES

A Special Report published by the editors of HEALTHY *Years* in conjunction with

UCLA Health

9

EASY EXERCISES
WALKING

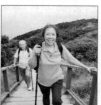

THE STAY FIT SERIES

A Special Report published by the editors of HEALTHY *Years* in conjunction with

UCLA Health

1. Easy Exercises for Aerobic Fitness

Cardio fitness is another term for aerobic exercise, the act of elevating your heart rate to boost cardiovascular performance and endurance. You can achieve peak aerobic fitness in a variety of heart-healthy ways. Our *Aerobic Fitness* guide describes how to safely engage in these fun and challenging activities—and explains the many ways they benefit your health.

2. Easy Exercises for Balance & Mobility

An antidote for the potentially dire result of falling down, *Easy Exercises for Balance & Mobility* describes the connection between balance and mobility, and offers exercises and specific information on how to build up crucial muscles for upper-body and lower-body strength. It also delves into the critical need for flexibility and how to achieve it without injury. Improving your balance and mobility is key to life-long independence. Just a few of these exercises a day can help.

3. Easy Exercises for Bones & Joints

As we get older, our bones and joints are not what they used to be, but we can maintain our strength and power by taking proper care of them. The key to a healthy exercise program is to get started and, then, to keep it up, making it a regular part of your life. Avoiding injury is crucial to these goals, and it often comes down to maintaining function and alleviating pain in our complex system of joints. *Bones & Joints* is intended to help you stay ahead of fitness-robbing injuries so you'll live to play again.

4. Easy Exercises for Core Fitness

Some of the most important muscles in the body are those in the hips, pelvis, abdomen, and trunk—otherwise known as "the core." And make no mistake: We use our core in every aspect of daily life. In *Core Fitness*, you'll learn the most beneficial types of core exercises and how to plan a routine, from exercises that involve free weights and dumbbells to others that use stability balls and resistance bands.

5. Easy Exercises for Flexibility

Cardio, core, and strength training, while important, don't complete the total fitness picture. Don't overlook the importance of proper warm-up and stretching, a key ingredient for better balance, and protection from injuries that can derail our quality of life. Our *Easy Exercises for Flexibility* guide describes the proper way to do static and dynamic stretching and deal with muscle soreness, as well as how to avoid injury, and more. Good flexibility is key to conducting all other exercises properly.

6. Easy Exercises for Strength & Power

Don't be intimidated by the thought of building and toning muscle. Our *Strength & Power* guide isn't about training for bodybuilding competitions. Rather, it discusses weight and resistance training for any age—always with safety first—using free weights, dumbbells, medicine and stability balls, resistance bands, weight machines, and more. Many of these exercises can be done at home as well as in a gym.

7. Easy Exercises for More Strength & Power

To maintain peak muscle efficiency, it's important to periodically advance your exercise routine. With *More Strength & Power*, you'll be able to create a program that focuses on the areas you need it most, and then change it as you progress. In this report, you'll find 55 exercises and 15 programs for your upper body, core, and lower body that will help keep you fit and in the prime of your life.

8. Easy Exercises: 10 Activities for Fitness & Fun

For some, climbing onto that treadmill and doing 30 or 45 minutes a few times a week can become a chore. Fortunately, there are myriad ways to stay fit while having fun along the way. Popular alternatives such as yoga, tai chi, qigong, water workouts, and dance are front and center in *10 Activities for Fitness & Fun*, which not only will remind you that fitness should be fun, but it just may be your inspiration.

9. Easy Exercises: Walking

There's more to walking for exercise than putting one foot in front of the other. In *Walking*, you'll learn about multiple styles—from speed walking to Nordic to walking for mindfulness—along with a surprising number of other factors, from motivation, goal-setting, and injury prevention to weather protection, road safety, proper footwear, and more.

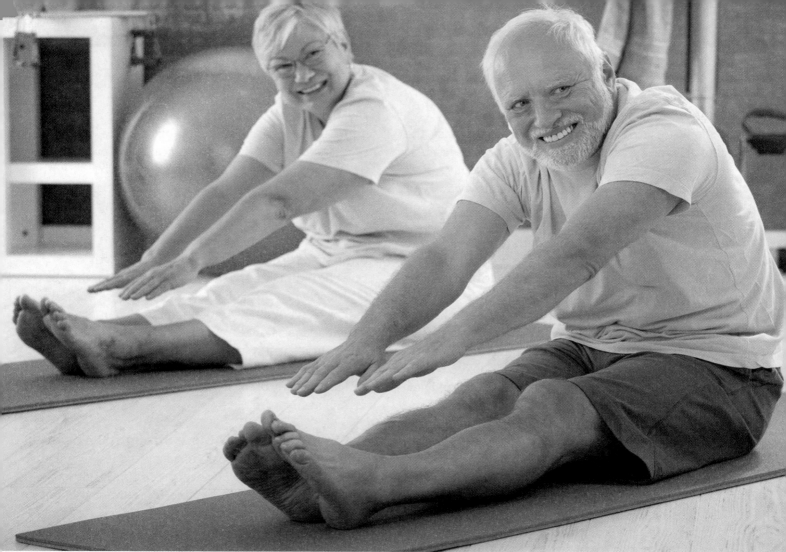

Staying physically active every day can help increase flexibility as you age.

1 The Flexibility Advantage

For the next few minutes, try to forget everything you've heard about flexibility. Suspend any preconceived notions about stretching, warming up, joint range of motion, and preventing injuries.

Just hit the reset button on the whole topic and let's start over with what evidence-based medicine tells us and common-sense practice shows us. It will affect almost every move you make for the rest of your life.

First off, what is flexibility? What happens to muscles and joints when we stretch? How does flexibility, or the lack of it, affect us right now? And why does flexibility often get overlooked in the information glut associated with aerobic fitness, strength, balance, and mobility in middle-aged and older adults?

Beyond Definitions

The answer to the first question is easy. Flexibility is the range of motion through which a joint moves, such as the neck, shoulders, elbow, spine, hip, knee, and ankles. This also includes the surrounding muscles, ligaments, and tendons, all of which work together with the joints to enable you to bend, stretch, twist, reach, lift, rotate, squat, walk, and climb with minimal effort.

But the degree of flexibility varies widely with the person and their joints. The shoulder joint is by far the most flexible joint in the body. For example, it can move your arm toward your body, away from the body, up, down, across, back, and around in a circle. Other joints can't do as much.

The flexibility of joints is affected by some behaviors you can change (physical activity, posture, and treatment of orthopaedic conditions, for example) and others you cannot (the structure of the joint, the pliability and length of the connective tissue, and your age). A study in Clinical Biomarkers found that increased range of motion after stretching could not be attributed to changes in the muscle-tendon unit, but might be due to increased stretching tolerance (see, "Increased Range Of Motion After Static Stretching May Result from Greater Tolerance To Stretching").

What Happens When A Muscle Is Stretched?

When you think about flexibility and stretching, you automatically think of muscles. After all, when you move and stretch, you feel it in your muscles. And when you are tight, your muscles are

RESEARCH FINDING

Increased Range Of Motion After Static Stretching May Result from Greater Tolerance To Stretching

Static stretching is known to increase range of motion, but little is known about what happens to the muscle-tendon unit. Researchers enrolled 49 volunteers and assigned them to stretching or control groups. The average range of motion increased in the stretching group, but the basic structure and length of the tendons and muscles remained the same. The increased range of motion could not be explained by structural changes, and was likely due to nerve-related, increased stretch tolerance of the subjects.

Clinical Biomechanics

often the first to tell you with a sudden twinge or soreness.

A muscle consists of multiple layers. From inside-out, the layers begin with small fibers (myofibers) surrounded by connective tissue (endomysium). Between 20 and 80 muscle fibers are grouped together in a bundle (fascicle) encapsulated by a thicker tissue called the perimysium. A muscle, as we recognize it, is formed by many fascicles within an external sheath called the epimysium (fascia), which connects to or becomes the tendon (see, "Anatomy Of A Muscle").

Anatomy of a Muscle

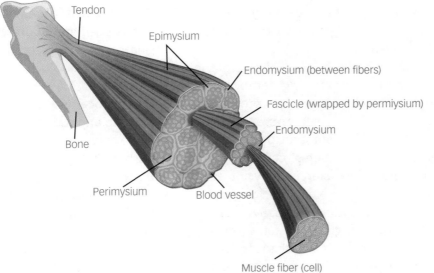

Tendon
Epimysium
Endomysium (between fibers)
Fascicle (wrapped by permiysium)
Endomysium
Bone
Perimysium
Blood vessel
Muscle fiber (cell)

© Dorling Kindersley | Thinkstock

Muscle fibers are surrounded by multiple layers of muscle tissue.

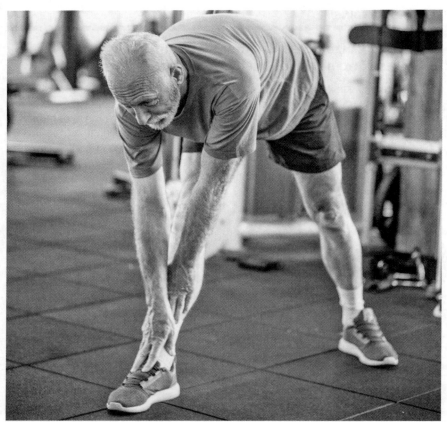

© Euroleadergroup121 | Dreamstime

Always stretch after warming up, never before.

What's In It for You?

Flexibility exercises like stretching and range-of-motion movements seem like the common-sense move, but many people, especially older adults, ignore their flexibility, or do exercises incorrectly, or at the wrong time, like before workouts, or do not perform them on a regular basis, so their flexibility never improves.

However, strong evidence shows that stretching and range-of-motion movements increase flexibility. The loss of flexibility can be prevented and at least partially restored by stretching. The evidence is even more compelling that a long-term stretching program can result in sustained increase in range of motion.

Improving your flexibility has a wide range of benefits. It can help you stay active longer and reduce your risk of common age-related physical ailments like strains and sprains.

Good flexibility keeps your muscles and joints strong and supple so you can continue to live a long, independent life. You will find it easier to perform everyday tasks and with less effort. For example, you need to be flexible to:

- Walk
- Climb stairs
- Get out of bed or a chair
- Get dressed and undressed
- Get in and out of a bathtub
- Bathe
- Lift objects
- Carry groceries
- Get into and out of a vehicle
- Drive a vehicle
- Turn your upper body
- Exercise
- Work in the yard
- Look over your shoulder
- Make a bed
- Tie your shoes
- Reach for an item a few feet away

Flexibility also helps you continue to enjoy your favorite sports and activities,

So how do your muscles affect flexibility? When a muscle is lengthened during a stretch or certain types of range-of-motion exercises, it's not only muscle tissues and components that are affected, but also the fibrous tissue (fascia), ligaments (that connect bones to bones), and tendons (that connect muscles to bones). Flexibility training can have an effect on all three in the short term.

Although the science of stretching is complex, stretching temporarily makes muscles longer. It is prescribed by physicians, recommended by physical therapists, and practiced by exercisers and athletes in almost every sport. But most exercise physiologists now say that the elongation process is temporary. Muscles eventually return to their normal length. What some forms of stretching might do is raise the tolerance level at which a person feels tightness or pain during a stretch, exercise, or sport-related activity.

like running, walking, golf, tennis, and swimming, and just enjoying an active life.

Flexibility and Age

As you may have noticed, flexibility decreases with age. The exact age varies from person to person, but 50 is often the age at which people noticeably begin to lose flexibility. It may happen sooner, maybe later, but it's going to happen unless you do something about it.

The warnings signs can be subtle at first, but then begin to worsen. You might have noticed that it's harder to bend or twist, as in turning to see if an automobile is approaching from the side or back. You may find it more difficult to get dressed or undressed, as in pulling off or putting on a sweater, shirt, or pullover. It might become harder to swing a golf club, tennis racket, or some other piece of sports equipment. You may even develop nagging muscle strains or joint sprains more often than when you were younger.

"Joint motion becomes more restricted and flexibility decreases because of changes in tendons and ligaments," says the American Academy of Orthopaedic Surgeons (AAOS). "The water content of tendons decreases as we age. This makes the tissues stiffer and less able to tolerate stress."

Another way to look at it is that parts of your body are like a rubber band. A new one stretches and then quickly snaps back to its original shape. Yet, over time the band loses its elasticity, can't stretch as far, or recoil fully.

Your body's muscle tissues are similar to that. After decades of use and poor body mechanics, they become like a worn out rubber band.

But the effects of these physical changes don't have to happen right now. There are ways to maintain or regain a full range of motion in some or all of your joints. A statement from the American Academy of Orthopaedic Surgeons (AAOS) says that much of the decline associated with aging is due to inactivity, not aging (see "Being Physically Active May Significantly Delay Or Minimize the Effects Of Aging").

Other studies suggest that middle-aged and older adults can improve range of motion in the neck, shoulders, elbows, wrists, hip, knees, and ankles when certain types of flexibility exercises, including some stretches, are performed over a period of time. The AAOS says that stretching is an excellent way to help maintain joint flexibility.

Specific attention paid to stretching, according to the Cleveland Clinic, can improve flexibility in middle-aged and older adults. Increasing flexibility can make you feel younger and more energized, improve your posture, and help reduce risks for injury. When combined with a cardiovascular and strength-training regimen, flexibility exercises can help you maintain or improve overall fitness.

Flexibility and Balance

Stretching through a full range of motion also helps maintain balance. As people age, coordination and balance enhances mobility and reduces the risk of falls.

The American College of Sports Medicine (ACSM) says that the two parts of fitness that are often overlooked are flexibility and balance. Both can play a vital role in overall function and fitness. When you are flexible you are lighter on your feet, more limber, and move with greater fluidity. You stand taller and for longer periods of time. Greater flexibility also increases your muscle control, which facilitates your coordination.

RESEARCH FINDING

Being Physically Active May Significantly Delay Or Minimize the Effects Of Aging

Research on senior athletes suggests that comprehensive fitness and nutrition routines help minimize bone and joint health decline and maintain overall physical health. An increasing amount of evidence demonstrates that age-related decline in the musculoskeletal system can be lessened, and that much of the deterioration associated with aging can be attributed to sedentary lifestyles instead of aging itself. Comprehensive fitness includes flexibility and balance. Two or more days a week of flexibility training, including sustained stretches and static/non-ballistic movements, are strongly recommended.

Journal of the American Academy of Orthopaedic Surgeons

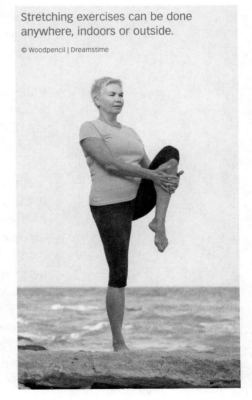

Stretching exercises can be done anywhere, indoors or outside.

© Woodpencil | Dreamstime

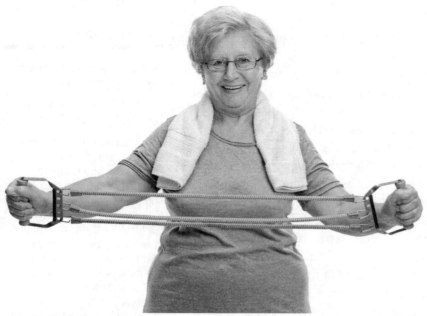
© Ljupco Smokovski | Dreamstime

Resistance bands are a great tool for building strength.

Flexibility and Strength

Can increased flexibility make you stronger? Research is inconclusive, but experts support the idea that the more range of motion a joint has, the longer the muscles surrounding that joint will be flexible, and therefore the more they can contract. In other words, increasing flexibility can allow your muscles to move within their full (or nearly full) range of motion. This can help muscles grow bigger and stronger during strength training.

The findings regarding the effects of strength training on flexibility are encouraging, but also mixed. A study in the *Journal of Strength and Conditioning* found that carefully constructed strength-training exercises can improve flexibility as effectively as static stretching (stretching a muscle and holding it for a short period of time) routines used in conditioning programs.

A recent study published in *Medicine & Science in Sports & Exercise* compared the results of strength and flexibility training to flexibility-only exercises in men between the ages of 50 and 74. The flexibility-only group increased its range of motion in shoulder abduction (raising the upper arms up to the side and away from the body) to a significantly greater extent than the strength and flexibility subjects. The findings suggest that, although strength (resistance) training is important for older men, flexibility training alone has a better chance of improving shoulder range of motion, if that is the goal.

However, research presented at a meeting of the ACSM showed that a scientifically constructed, full-range resistance training regimen can improve flexibility, as well as typical static stretching.

The message to remember regarding flexibility and strength is that both should be addressed in a fitness program for middle-aged and older

Research appears to back it up. University of Minnesota exercise scientists say that flexibility exercises can improve overall ease of movement, decrease stress on the joints, and reduce risk of injury, especially from falls. A study in the *Journal of Sports Science & Medicine* found that hip-joint mobility was positively associated with balance ability and the risk of falls in older adults.

Flexibility and Circulation

Flexibility-related activities increase the amount of blood that flows to the muscles. This blood flow brings nutrients and removes waste products that have accumulated in muscle tissue. Improved circulation can help reduce the amount of time it takes to recover after an injury to a muscle.

Another benefit to good circulation: It can help protect you against a host of illnesses, from diabetes to kidney disease to cardiovascular disease.

In fact, people age 40 and older who performed well on a sit-and-reach test (a seated forward bend that measures flexibility; see page 25) had less stiffness in their arterial walls, an indicator of their risk for stroke and heart attack, according to the *American Journal of Physiology*.

adults. The ACSM recommends strength training two to three times per week on alternate days.

Flexibility and Rehabilitation

In the midst of all the controversy regarding the benefits and risks of stretching, the health-care community seems to agree that range of motion and/or passive stretching should be incorporated into almost every program of rehabilitation for muscle and joint injuries and conditions.

The great advantage of supervised rehabilitation is that the person who needs it has a trained physical or occupational therapist who can select appropriate, individual-specific strength and flexibility exercises.

Flexibility and Massage

Most people would agree that a massage feels good and makes them feel better even though evidence that it enhances long-term flexibility is scarce. However, in the short-term, massage can reduce pain, increase circulation, reduce muscle tension, and improve range of motion.

Cochrane Summaries concluded that massage might be beneficial for patients with low back pain that lasts four to 12 weeks, especially when combined with education and exercise. Other studies have found that massage (or, specifically, soft tissue manipulation) "promotes improvement in muscle and joint motion." Still, massage cannot cure or reverse the course of a medical condition or disease.

An increasingly popular form of self-massage (self-myofascial release, SMR) during warm ups and cool downs for physical activity is the use of foam rollers or similar devices. The person moves muscle groups forward and backward against the roller, using the weight of the body to create pressure.

More than a dozen studies on the topic have been published, with mixed results. One study using a tennis ball instead of a foam roller found that SMR improved scores on a sit-and-reach test (see "Self-Myofascial Release May Increase Hamstring and Lumbar Spine Flexibility"). Other investigations have yielded conflicting results on the immediate effects of SMR on hip flexion (no effect), knee flexion (limited positive effect), and ankle flexion (limited positive effect). Of the five additional studies involving the sit-and-reach test, self-myofascial release produced positive results in three, but no effect in the other two.

Why Now?

If flexibility is that vital to perform so many activities of daily living, why haven't we heard more about it? Probably because we take it for granted and perhaps because loss of flexibility comes on gradually. We only take notice when it begins to decline and affects our daily life.

Heart attacks and strokes can be dramatic events, which often motivate people to make drastic lifestyle changes. Loss of flexibility is insidious, even sneaky, and it's not an emergency. Emergency rooms are not filled with people who have lost flexibility. Sadly, many older adults just let it happen by being sedentary and not being proactive about their bone, muscle, and joint health. By taking some decidedly undramatic steps now (meaning flexibility exercises

RESEARCH FINDING

Self-Myofascial Release May Increase Hamstring and Lumbar Spine Flexibility

British researchers designed a study to determine if using a tennis ball as a self-myofascial release (SMR) device would have an effect on flexibility. Twenty-four men were assigned to an experimental group that used the technique on the bottom (plantar) aspect of the foot or to a control group. The result was a significant increase in flexibility of the hamstrings and lumbar spine among those who used SMR. Other studies have been inconclusive.

Journal of Bodywork and Movement Therapies

Foam rollers are an increasingly popular form of self-massage.

© Ihor Bulyhin | Dreamstime

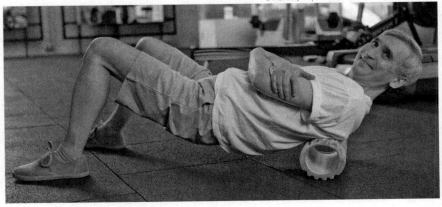

Static Stretching May Impair Lower Body Strength and Performance

Researchers studied 17 young men to determine the effect of passive static stretching on the lower body musculature and strength before performing a demanding exercise. They noted a significant decrease in lower body strength and stability immediately following the passive static stretch as measured by barbell and free-weight squats. The study suggests that intensive stretching should be avoided before training the lower body or performing certain exercises in favor of a dynamic warm-up using resistance training equipment.

Journal of Strength and Conditioning Research

and activities), you can ensure that lack of flexibility doesn't cause your world to get smaller as you age.

The Truth About Stretching

Stretching and range-of-motion exercises and movements are the best ways to improve flexibility. You probably think of stretching when you think of flexibility. Proper stretching is essential to increase flexibility, but only if it is done correctly. The whole topic of stretching continues to be a moving target. There are lots of ways to stretch, some of them safe and useful, others unsafe and either unproductive or counterproductive. Here is a look at the types of stretching and which ones you should do, and avoid.

Static Stretching

As previously mentioned, static stretching is assuming a stretch position and holding it for a short period of time. If you do it by yourself, it's called active

Warming Up Should Not Be Limited To Stretching Exercises

Exercisers who warm up by only stretching will not benefit from it and may experience a decrease in performance, according to a Scandinavian study. Researchers used an analysis of multiple studies to estimate the effects of pre-exercise static stretching on strength, power, and explosive muscular performance. More than 100 studies (over a period of four decades) involving thousands of exercisers revealed that using static stretches as the only activity during a warm-up routine should be avoided. Although the goal of most recreational and fitness exercisers is not muscular performance, the study reinforces other findings that stress the need for a balanced approach to warming up.

Scandinavian Journal of Medicine & Science in Sports

stretching; with a partner to assist, it's passive stretching. This is the type of stretching with which most people are familiar and the style that is considered one of the most effective for older adults. (Static stretching is the foundation for many of the stretching routines outlined in Chapter 4.) It is also done after a proper warm up or after completing a sport or activity when the muscles and body are warmed up.

However, you should never do static stretching before an activity or workout. Not only can it increase your risk of strain and injury since the muscles are not properly warmed up, it may hinder your exercise performance. In fact, among athletes, static stretching has been found to decrease power and speed, at least for the first few minutes after stretching (see, "Static Stretching May Impair Lower Body Strength and Performance").

Dynamic Stretching

Dynamic stretching is moving the body or parts of the body without holding a stretch position. Dynamic stretching, according to the editors of the *Encyclopedia of Sports Medicine*, results in a durable rebalancing of muscle strength, flexibility, and stiffness, and does not damage ligaments.

Dynamic stretching also can be used as a proper warm-up before exercise, including flexibility exercises. The importance of warming up before strenuous physical activity or sports performance is supported by decades of evidence. It improves performance and prevents injuries (see "Warming Up Should Not Be Limited To Stretching Exercises").

The goal of warming up is to increase circulation and the temperature of the muscles. One of the most dangerous ways to injure a muscle is to stretch it as far as it will go before warming up.

The most sensible and practical way

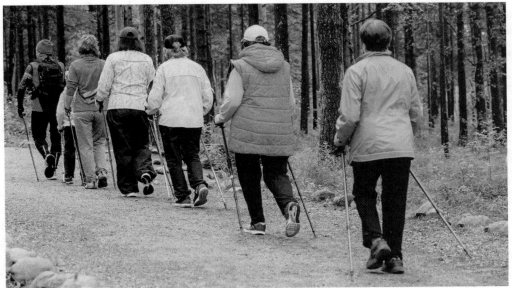
Exercising can be more fun when in a group!

© John1300 | Dreamstime

Warming Up To Walk

Many older adults prefer walking as their choice of physical activity, and it's a good one. How do you warm up for walking? By walking. Slowly at first, then at a pace fast enough to get your heart into its target zone, while at the same time enhancing lower body flexibility.

If you want to include flexibility exercises before walking, Foot/Ankle Circles (Exercise #3), Leg Swings (Exercise #19), and Arm Circles (Exercise #47, all in Chapter 3) are safe and help to increase circulation and muscle temperature.

to stretch dynamically is by replicating the movements you will use in the physical activity to follow. Tennis players who warm up by hitting easy groundstrokes, volleys, and serves are a good example, assuming they gradually work in some quick starts and stops and short-distance runs into their warm-up routines. Golfers who go through their repertoire of shots on the driving range accomplish the same goal.

Besides replicating specific activity movements, brisk walking, light jogging, using an elliptical machine, slow-paced cycling on a stationary bike, or light calisthenics like jumping jacks and standing leg lifts can help you break a sweat, gradually elevate the heart rate, and increase circulation (see "Warming Up To Walk").

Research supports the use of dynamic stretching to improve the quality of static stretching and thus overall flexibility. A study in the *Journal of Sports Science & Medicine* found that the combination of dynamic and static stretching improved flexibility between 36.3 and 85.6 percent among 25 subjects.

Used together—dynamic stretching warm-ups followed by static stretching exercises—is the best way to reduce risk of injury and improve overall flexibility.

PNF Stretching

Another type of stretching is proprioceptive neuromuscular facilitation (PNF), which is an effective way to increase range of motion, although there is a limited amount of research that explains how it works.

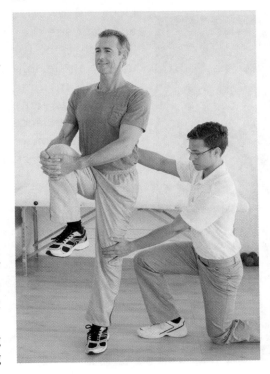

© Wavebreakmedia Ltd | Thinkstock

PNF stretching is performed under the guidance of a licensed therapist and may help improve your range of motion.

PNF stretching increases flexibility in athletes

Researchers in Greece and Italy tested 18 gymnasts to determine the effects of three warm-up methods of stretching—static, PNF, and stretching exercises performed on a vibration platform. Flexibility was assessed with a sit-and-reach test, jumping, and counter-jumping movements immediately after and again 15 minutes after stretching. Significant differences in flexibility were observed after all three stretching methods, but PNF stretching increased flexibility at a higher level than the other methods 15 minutes after the exercises were performed.

The Journal of Sports Medicine and Physical Fitness

Repeat resistance exercises 2 to 3 times a week on nonconsecutive days.

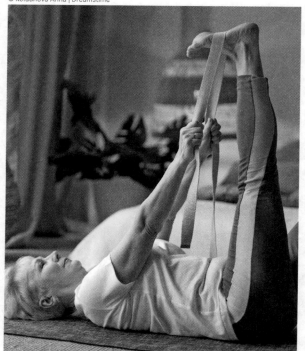

© Koldunova Anna | Dreamstime

PNF is used more in clinical and rehabilitation settings, as well as for elite exercisers and athletes, than in everyday use. It was originally developed to treat neuromuscular conditions, such as polio and multiple sclerosis.

There are several ways to perform PNF stretches, but all of them involve some combination of stretching a muscle to its limit, then contracting, holding, and/or relaxing it. Specific sequences, usually conducted with a partner, include "contract-relax," "hold-relax," and "hold-relax-contract." PNF stretches can be modified so that a person can stretch without a partner.

A study in the *Journal of Human Kinetics* reported that when PNF is performed consistently and post-exercise, it increases athletic performance, range of motion, muscular strength, and power. An article in *The Journal of Sports Medicine and Physical Fitness* found that PNF stretching used during warm-ups increased flexibility in competitive gymnasts (see "PNF Stretching Increases Flexibility In Athletes").

The American College of Sports Medicine (ACSM) endorses PNF stretches, along with dynamic and static stretches, as effective for improving flexibility. Keep in mind that PNF is done under the guidance and supervision of a licensed therapist. However, it can be taught so you can do it on your own, if desired.

Ballistic Stretching

Unless you are an elite athlete, the one kind of stretching to avoid is called ballistic. Ballistic stretches involve rapid, bouncing movement that moves the joint beyond its normal range of motion or a range of motion limited by muscle tightness.

Ballistic stretching can cause injury and soreness, and it doesn't allow enough time for the muscles to adapt to the stretch. Instead of relaxing the muscle, it increases tension and makes it hard to stretch the surrounding connective tissues. Bottom line: no bouncing.

Stretching and Injuries

Although stretching has been promoted to prevent injuries, the research does not support this theory. Stretching immediately before exercise does not appear to prevent overuse or acute injuries. But no one disputes that warming up before strenuous physical activity lessens the risk of injury, so dynamic stretching within the framework of warming up could indirectly prevent injuries or lessen the risk. Because flexibility exercises help improve blood flow to the muscles, stretching an injured muscle also may speed-up recovery.

Still, like any other type of exercise or movement, injuries are almost unavoidable. When you work to improve your flexibility, you may encounter common ailments like muscle soreness, strains, and sprains.

Muscle Soreness

Some muscle soreness is to be expected when beginning an exercise program, but it should resolve itself within a couple of days. You can minimize it by warming up properly, gradually increasing the intensity and duration of a stretch, and not overdoing it.

Strained (Pulled) Quadriceps

Quad injuries are among the most common, and the easiest to treat. The quadriceps are a group of four muscles in front of the upper leg that work together with the hamstrings (behind the upper leg) to extend and bend the leg.

A strained quadricep involves a partial or complete tear of one of those four muscles, or their tendons, when stretched beyond their normal limits. When the muscles are fatigued, overused, or not adequately warmed up, they are at increased risk of strain. An imbalance between weak quadriceps and stronger hamstrings can also cause the injury, as can simply having tight quadriceps.

Traditional treatment is rest and cold packs applied for 15 to 20 minutes, three to four times a day for the first 48 to 72 hours. After that, apply moist heat for the next 48- to 72-hour period, three to four times a day, followed by gentle stretching. Aspirin, ibuprofen, and naproxen may relieve pain and inflammation.

Strained (Pulled) Hamstring

The hamstring muscles are the three muscles that run down the back of the thigh. A cold (not properly warmed up) hamstring that is required to contract at maximum intensity is at high risk for injury.

You'll know if you've pulled a hamstring by the severe pain behind the upper leg or buttock, possible muscle spasms, bruising and tenderness, and swelling. Rest, ice applications, elevation, and compression wraps are first aid treatments. Aspirin, acetaminophen, ibuprofen, and naproxen may relieve the pain.

To reduce the risk of a pulled hamstring, gradually increase the stretch intensity, frequency, and duration from week to week. Stop exercising if you feel tightness in the back of your legs.

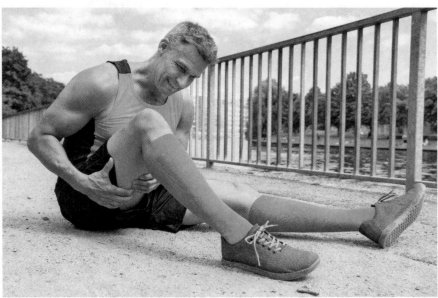

© Andrey Popov | Dreamstime

If you suffer an injury, see your doctor before continuing your exercise routine.

Strained (Pulled) Calf Muscle

The two large muscles in the back of the lower leg (soleus and gastrocnemius) are called calf muscles, and they are at risk every time you push off—even when walking. When the muscles are stretched beyond their normal capacity, the muscle fibers tear away from the tendon. Joggers, runners, and tennis players are particularly susceptible to strains.

The symptoms are sudden pain in the back of the lower leg between the knee and heel, pain when pushing off, stiffness, weakness, and bruising. Rest, ice, compression, elevation, and over-the-counter pain medications are the initial treatments.

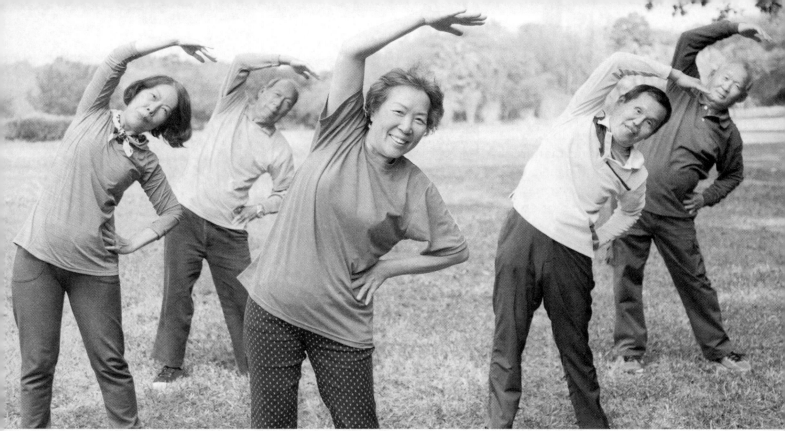

© Tom Wang | Dreamstime

Love the outdoors? Check with your local senior center or gym for outdoor classes.

2 Choices and Guidelines

Fitness programs, including those that have a flexibility component, are available in a variety of formats. They are in books, magazines, online, on DVDs, and at health clubs, churches, hospitals, colleges/universities, senior centers, YMCAs/YWCAs, golf and tennis clubs, municipal recreation departments, and neighborhood fitness centers.

Enroll in programs for groups or do your own program at home. Your problem won't be finding a program, but in choosing one that is right for you.

RESEARCH FINDING

Lack Of Motivation Cited As Factor In High Drop-Out Rate Among Older Women In Exercise Programs

A study found that about one-half of all women enrolled in aerobic exercise and resistance training programs failed to complete the classes. More than 200 women, average age 70, enrolled in a program designed to minimize the decline normally associated with aging. Fifty percent completed the aerobic training course; 56 percent finished the strength training sessions. Several factors were associated with the high drop-out rate, including lack of motivation.

Clinical Interventions in Aging

Sticking with the Program

The biggest problem with exercise programs is that too many people don't stick with them. A recent study showed that about half of older women who enrolled in programs dropped out (see "Lack Of Motivation Cited As Factor In High Drop-Out Rate Among Older Women In Exercise Programs").

One of the most important factors in choosing the right program—and sticking with it—is to know what you expect to get out of it. What are your goals with improved flexibility? Strength? Balance? Overall fitness? Prevention? All of the above?

All of those expectations are reasonable, but your chances of succeeding are better if you set a few modest, realistic goals, and keep track of your progress. Give your program time to work—weeks and months, not days.

A study in *Current Gerontology and Geriatrics Research* found that goal setting, among other factors, is beneficial in getting adults to adhere to exercise programs (see "Setting Goals Increases Adherence To Group Exercise Programs").

Finding a good program match is also more likely if you choose one that has built-in supervision and support (see "Supervision Helps Adults Adhere To Exercise Programs"). Doing flexibility exercises at home is quick and easy, but having an exercise partner or a group of exercisers with the same goals is more likely to become a good habit instead of a one-and-done experience.

Getting enjoyment and positive results significantly increases participation in physical activity, according to a survey of adults engaged in a National Council of Aging-approved program called Active Living Every Day (see "Active Living Every Day Program Improves Enjoyment Of Physical Activity").

Also "10 Ways To Stick with An Exercise Program" on page 20, is a composite list of all the factors, beginning with goal setting, support/supervision, enjoyment, and positive results, that make it more likely you won't quit. Adhering to a program and achieving your goals means you have made the right choice.

Choices

This special report, *Easy Exercises for Flexibility*, is one choice. Chapter 3 has 64 stretching exercises from which to choose, divided among three categories to offer all-around flexibility: lower body, trunk/core, and upper body. Chapter 5 offers sample flexibility workout programs to help you get going. And if you enroll in a group exercise program, use this book to supplement what you do and learn in a supervised program.

At wellness centers, clinics, or in your home, physical and occupational therapists can design and supervise individual flexibility programs that are appropriate for you. The advantages

Setting Goals Increases Adherence To Group Exercise Programs

A study of 63 adults, average age 64, found that goal-setting is an effective method of motivating older adults to adhere to a group exercise program. The participants were assigned to a six-week exercise group, followed by a five-week program that included motivational strategies, or to an exercise-only program. A third group of volunteers were assigned to a control group that did not participate in either the exercise or motivation group. The motivational components for the experimental group were instituted at various stages of the program. Exercise contracts, instructor feedback, self-monitoring, and exercise prompts were also beneficial in motivating older adults to adhere to an exercise program.

Current Gerontology and Geriatrics Research

RESEARCH FINDING

Supervision Helps Older Adults Adhere To Exercise Programs

Australian researchers reviewed nine studies to determine the factors associated with better adherence to exercise programs among older adults. Among the measurements used to track adherence were finishing a program, sessions attended, and the average number of home exercise routines completed per week. Adherence rates were higher in supervised sessions. Other predictors were higher socioeconomic status, living alone, fewer health conditions, taking fewer medications, and better cognitive ability.

Journal of Physiology

RESEARCH FINDING

Active Living Every Day Program Improves Enjoyment Of Physical Activity

Participation in a program approved by the National Council on Aging titled "Active Living Every Day" could be effective in helping adult workers become more active by enhancing their enjoyment of physical activity. Researchers offered the ALED classes to a control group and an intervention group, and used separate scales to rate how participants felt during physical activity, as well as their level of enjoyment as a result of the program. The subjects felt physically better after taking part in the ALED activities, which translated into increased physical activity, and they reported more enjoyment of physical activity after the program had been completed.

International Journal of Health Promotion and Education

are expertise, instruction, efficiency, accountability, supervision, and motivation.

The disadvantages are cost, lack of social interaction gained by working out with a group, and difficulty in finding qualified professionals who are knowledgeable. You also have to find someone with whom you are comfortable.

The rate of turnover among personal trainers is high. Look for someone who has made a career of working with people like you, rather than someone who is transitioning to another position or working as a personal trainer in his or her spare time. Get references and ask friends or family members for recommendations.

Another option is to participate in range-of-motion exercises that revolve around dynamic stretching. These include low-impact aerobics classes, yoga, tai chi, and Pilates.

Low-Impact Aerobics Classes

The best one-size-fits-all class for flexibility is a group aerobics class. The ultimate goal is aerobic (cardiovascular) fitness, but instructors and their students have to go through warm-up and flexibility exercises before getting to the aerobic component.

If you are a beginner or older adult not used to regular exercise, make sure you choose a class appropriate for your age and condition, and that your instructor knows your limitations.

Yoga

Yoga is a mind/body series of movements called asanas that combine stretching and controlled breathing to achieve relaxation and a stabilized mood. Its main purpose is not to improve range of motion or flexibility, but those attributes are clear benefits.

Yoga continues to gain in popularity, according to a report from the U.S. National Center for Health Statistics. More than 21 million American adults, including 3 percent of those age 65 and older, say they've tried yoga in the past year (see "Yoga Gaining In Popularity Among Americans").

For some people, yoga is an alternative or complementary exercise that promotes flexibility, strength, and endurance. For others, it is more of a spiritual experience. The general consensus is that yoga offers both physical and psychological benefits. The following is a summary of recent research, most of it yoga-positive, but not conclusive.

- Yoga may help reduce pain and improve function. — *National Center for Complementary and Integrative Health*
- Yoga results in moderate improvements for gait, balance, upper and lower body flexibility, lower body strength, and weight loss. — *Journal of Aging and Physical Activity*
- Yoga is effective in improving function and symptoms of chronic low back pain, but is no more effective than stretching. — *Archives of Internal Medicine*
- Yoga enhances muscular strength and body flexibility. — *International Journal of Yoga*

- Older adults are at higher risk of developing musculoskeletal problems, such as sprains and strains, when doing yoga. — *BMC Complementary and Alternative Medicine*, (see "Older Adults At Higher Risk Of Strains and Sprains In Some Yoga Poses").
- Yoga may be effective as an adjunct to address some medical conditions, but is not yet a proven stand-alone, curative treatment. — *Evidence-Based Complementary and Alternative Medicine*

Says one UCLA physical therapist, "Key yoga movements promote overall flexibility in multiple muscle groups and in a coordinated way, as opposed to just stretching single muscles and/or muscles groups. The results translate better to real life."

There are many varieties of yoga from which to choose based on your age, comfort level, and physical limitations. Many gyms offer "silver" yoga classes designed for older adults. Most integrate slow, gentle movements with a mixture of both standing and sitting poses.

Also, check with your local YMCA, community senior center, or even hospital. Most offer gentle or restorative yoga classes modified for seniors with physical limitations or that are less demanding than traditional yoga classes.

Hatha and Iyengar yoga are all-around styles adopted by many yoga studios and gym classes. These styles place a greater emphasis on proper body alignment and balance. They also rely on props such as straps, bolsters, and blocks to help with support and reduce the risk of strain or injury.

Certain yoga styles might be better suited for older adults. For instance, chair yoga, in which all the movements are practiced while sitting in or using a chair for support, is ideal if you have mobility or balance problems.

The case for yoga, as with all forms of exercise, depends on the needs,

goals, and the physical condition of the person. Its benefits have been widely promoted and occasionally backed by scientific evidence. For some people, the same benefits are available in other and less demanding forms of exercise, such as flexibility training, static stretching, and range-of-motion exercises.

Tai Chi

Studies have shown that tai chi can improve balance, lower the risk of falls, and provide a sense of well-being. Reputable health institutions associate tai chi with aerobic capacity, less joint pain, energy, and stamina, but the evidence regarding tai chi and flexibility is not as strong.

The study most frequently cited was conducted at Stanford and published in *Alternative Therapies in Health and Medicine*. The group comprised 39 women, average age 66, with below-average fitness and at least one cardiovascular risk factor, who took 36 tai chi classes over the course of 12 weeks. Tests showed significantly increased strength and flexibility in the upper and lower body.

However, since then, no major studies have associated tai chi with increased flexibility. A presentation at the annual scientific meeting of the American College of Rheumatology reported that tai

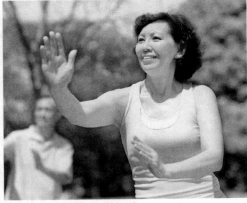

© Fuse | Thinkstock

The slow, gentle movements of tai chi can lower joint pain, increase energy and stamina, and may help less-mobile seniors improve their flexibility.

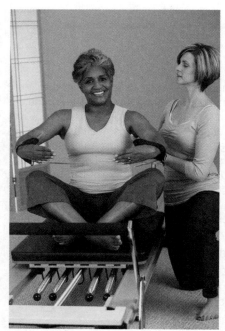
© Jon Feingersh | Thinkstock

Pilates uses range-of-motion movements to improve core strength and posture needed for better flexibility.

chi improved pain, fatigue, and stiffness caused by arthritis.

The National Center for Complementary and Integrative Health says, "In general, studies of tai chi have been small or they have had designs that may limit their conclusions. The cumulative evidence suggests that additional research is needed before tai chi can be widely recommended as an effective therapy."

That said, there remains some evidence that it is beneficial for some individuals and that it is safe. In this way, its slow, gentle movements may be an easy entry point for some older adults to begin range-of-motion exercise.

Keep in mind that people with the following conditions should consult a physician before beginning a tai chi program:

- osteoporosis
- chest pain with minimal exertion
- severe shortness of breath
- dizziness or fainting spells
- uncontrolled blood pressure
- gait and balance disorders

Pilates

Pilates is a program of low-impact strength and endurance movements designed to increase core strength for better posture, balance, and flexibility. Most of the movements can be done on the floor or a mat, or specialized designed machines called reformers. These consist of a platform that moves back and forth along a carriage and straps to help execute and support movements. Programs can be individualized for beginners or seasoned exercisers.

Because Pilates is not aerobic exercise, it should be combined with other activities that get the heart rate into its target zone and keep it there for 10 to 30 minutes per session. The Centers for Disease Control and Prevention recommends 150 minutes of moderate aerobic activity or 75 minutes of vigorous aerobic per week.

Still, Pilates, like yoga, can offer range-of-motion movements that can improve flexibility. Pilates places a greater emphasis on strengthening the core compared to yoga, and helps to improve posture, both of which are key to greater flexibility. This is one reason Pilates is so popular among professional dancers, who rely on the practice to keep them limber and mobile.

A study in the *Journal of Strength & Conditioning Research* suggested that people can improve their muscular endurance and flexibility using relatively low-intensity Pilates exercises that do not require equipment or a high degree of skill, and are easy to master.

BMC Medical Research Methodology used a review of studies to determine that there was inconclusive evidence that Pilates was effective in reducing low back pain. There was no mention of flexibility.

A study in *Geriatric Rehabilitation* concluded that older adults may benefit from Pilates-based exercises that are integrated into traditional resistance and balance training programs.

A study of low back therapy found that Pilates offers equivalent improvements to massage therapy and other forms of exercise therapy (see "Pilates Offers Short-Term Improvement In Low Back Pain Equal To Other Forms Of Exercise"). The implication is that the

RESEARCH FINDING

Pilates Offers Short-Term Improvement In Low Back Pain Equal To Other Forms Of Exercise

A review of 14 randomized controlled trials was conducted to evaluate the effectiveness of Pilates exercise in people with chronic low back pain. Pilates provided significant improvement in pain and functional ability (presumably including flexibility) compared to usual care and physical activity for a period of 4-15 weeks, but not at 24 weeks. No consistent differences in improvements were found between Pilates, massage therapy, or other forms of exercise. Therefore, Pilates was as effective as other exercise methods, at least for the short term. Some patients with chronic low back pain may benefit from Pilates exercise more than others.
PLOS One

improvement would involve increased flexibility.

Pilates is not recommended for people who have unstable blood pressure, a risk of blood clots, severe osteoporosis, or a herniated disc. Check with your doctor if you are not sure before enrolling in a Pilates course or class.

Do They Help?

Each of these range-of-motion exercises have proven to be beneficial for certain individuals and physical conditions over extended periods of time. But keep in mind that what works for one person is not necessarily as effective for others.

In light of current research that indicates flexibility exercises and stretches should be task- or activity-specific, it is fair to ask how each of these exercise forms will help people—especially middle-aged and older adults—perform the normal activities of daily life. Does holding a yoga position, assuming a tai chi pose, or performing a Pilates exercise help you reach something on the top shelf, get up and out of a chair, or get into, drive, and get out of a car? If they do, then they might be the right choice of flexibility exercise for you. If not, there are other ways to safely achieve flexibility goals.

Stretching Guidelines

Doctor- or physical therapist-approved range-of-motion exercises and static or dynamic stretches are all acceptable ways to maintain or improve flexibility. Just as with other forms of exercise, you need to follow certain guidelines and parameters to ensure safety and make sure you gain the most benefits from your flexibility workout routines (see "Eight Times Not To Stretch").

When?

Regardless of the time of day you choose to perform flexibility exercises, don't stretch first. Warm up to loosen up, to raise muscle temperature, and to increase circulation. Then begin your flexibility exercise routine.

By preference or necessity, many people exercise in the mornings. It becomes part of their daily routine and helps them get ready for the rest of the day. Others find that exercising later in the day is more relaxing. If you have time, do both—a few minutes in the morning, and a few minutes in the late afternoon or evening.

Stretching and/or doing range-of-motion exercises during the workday is effective for relieving physical and mental stress. Workplace exercises (see Chapter 4) can be performed at a desk, computer, or workstation. If you are new to a flexibility routine, begin your program in the morning. Add other sessions as your body needs them and as your schedule allows.

How Often?

The American College of Sports Medicine (ACSM) says to perform flexibility exercises at least two to three days a week. Eventually, as you improve your flexibility and stretching routines become more of a habit, you could increase the frequency to every day, if desired. However, in the beginning, stick with the ACSM's recommendation and with a day off in between workouts. Also, do not worry if you occasionally skip a day or two. Daily flexibility training is beneficial, but you won't lose flexibility gains that quickly.

How Far?

When you perform static stretching, hold the stretch to a point of resistance, but not to a point of pain. If you go too far with a stretch, you won't be able to hold it for long and you'll risk an injury. And again, never do any ballistic or "bouncing" stretches.

How Long?

The ACSM recommends that each stretch should be held for 10 to 30

Eight Times Not To Stretch

If you have any doubts about the appropriateness of an exercise or stretching program, consult a physician who has a background in exercise, fitness, or sports medicine. Unless you have been instructed otherwise, don't stretch:

1. If you have a joint that is not stable or is overly lax.
2. If you have certain vascular diseases or conditions.
3. If you have had recent surgery.
4. If you have suffered a recent muscle strain or joint sprain.
5. If you have recently suffered a fractured bone.
6. If you have osteoporosis.
7. If you have acute pain on movement.
8. If there is inflammation in the area of a joint that will be involved.

ACSM Ranks Top 20 Fitness Trends

Each year, the American College of Sports Medicine (ACSM) ranks the top 20 fitness trends. The rankings are based on responses to an electronic survey of thousands of fitness and exercise professionals around the world. Although the term "core fitness" does not appear as a stand-alone trend, it is incorporated in more than half of the 20 programs. The top 20 are:

1. Wearable technology
2. High-intensity interval training
3. Group training*
4. Free-weight training*
5. Personal training*
6. Exercise Is Medicine (EIM)
7. Body weight training*
8. Fitness programs for older adults*
9. Health/wellness coaching
10. Using fitness professionals
11. Exercise for weight loss
12. Functional fitness training*
13. Outdoor activities
14. Yoga*
15. Licensure for fitness professionals
16. Lifestyle medicine
17. Circuit training*
18. Worksite well-being programs*
19. Outcome measurements*
20. Children and exercise

* Programs that may include elements of core training

Health and Fitness Journal

seconds. There is no research that says holding a position for a minute is more beneficial than holding a stretch for 30 seconds. You can even break the 30 seconds into three 10-second repetitions, if needed.

How Many Repetitions?

Repetitions depend on the type of stretching exercise. They can range from two to 10. Make sure to follow the recommended number of reps for each exercise.

How Many Exercises?

There is no perfect number. For those who need a general flexibility program, two or three stretching exercises for each major area of the body—lower body, core/trunk, and upper body—is the goal. In other words, Between six and nine stretches per session, divided among the lower body, core, and upper body. The sample workouts highlighted in Chapter 5 are based on this criteria and include a total of eight stretches per program.

Not a Complete Package

A flexibility program that includes static stretching routines and range-of-motion movements do not comprise a complete exercise program. It will not directly increase your cardiovascular fitness, strength, or power, which is why you need to complement your flexibility exercises with aerobic and strength training routines to ensure all-around fitness.

Avoid Common Mistakes

Here are some mistakes to avoid when beginning a flexibility program:

▶ **Don't static stretch first.** Always warm up with dynamic stretching, then go into your static stretches. This is especially important early in the morning when you have been inactive for many hours.

▶ **Don't bounce or bob.** Stretch and hold for 10 to 30 seconds.
▶ **Don't stretch an injured muscle** unless you are working with a physical therapist.
▶ **Don't ignore problem areas.** Older adults often have tight hamstrings, for example. Make sure your flexibility routine covers your entire body.
▶ **Don't go too fast.** Slow down, take your time, take a break between stretches.
▶ **Don't hold your breath** while performing a stretch.

Flex Tests: How Flexible Are You?

Before you begin a flexibility program, it is a good idea to gauge your current level of flexibility. This way you can target problem areas that may need extra attention, and help you measure your progress.

Testing for flexibility can be complex or simple. Exercise scientists and physical therapists use instruments called goniometers to measure degrees of joint rotation at the extremes of range of motion. Flexibility is joint-specific, according to the authors of the *Exercise Testing and Prescription Lab Manual* (Human Kinetics). Determining the range of motion for one joint is not an indicator of flexibility in other joints.

The simplest and least scientific way to measure flexibility is how a person performs activities of daily living. If you can flex and extend a joint, reach, turn, twist, kneel, climb stairs, and bend with relative ease, the joint is flexible.

Between those scientific and simple tests are a few flexibility self-tests you can do at home. They are strictly informal, do-it-yourself measurements that will give you a general idea of your current flexibility. Be careful, do them slowly, don't hurt yourself, and don't do them at all if there is the slightest risk of injury.

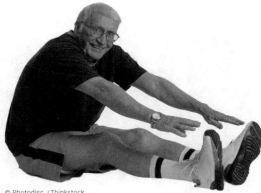

© Photodisc | Thinkstock

The sit-and-reach test is a general measure of lower body flexibility.

Lower Body: Sit-And-Reach

1. Sit on the floor with your legs stretched outward.
2. Keeping your back flat and not rounded, bend forward at the hips.
3. Reach toward your toes. Do not bounce or stretch to the point of pain.
4. Note the distance from the tips of the middle fingers to the top of your toes.
5. If you can reach past your toes, you have above-average lower body flexibility.
6. If you can touch your toes, you have average lower body flexibility.
7. If you cannot touch your toes, or need to bend your knees to touch them, you have below-average lower body flexibility.

Hips, Buttocks:
Lying Knee-To-Chest

1. Lie on your back and draw your knees to your chest.
2. Continue holding the left knee in that position while you extend the right leg until it lies flat on the floor.

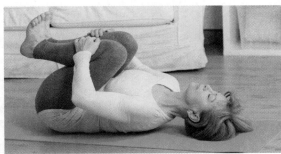

© KatarzynaBialasiewicz | Thinkstock

The lying knee-to-chest test can help to measure hip flexibility.

3. Repeat the movement with the other leg.
4. If you cannot completely extend one leg while bringing the opposite knee to within a few inches of your chest, your hip flexors and buttocks may be too tight.

Lower Back, Hamstrings:
Standing Toe Reach

Note: Do not perform this test if you have any question regarding the condition of your back.

1. Stand with your feet together, knees straight but not locked.
2. Bend forward and reach for the floor. Try to keep your back flat.
3. Your lower back and hamstring flexibility is good if you can touch or nearly touch your toes with little effort and no discomfort.
4. If you can't come close, you may be susceptible to lower back injuries.

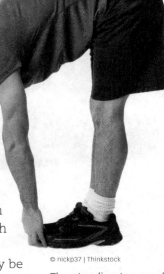

© nickp37 | Thinkstock

The standing toe reach tests lower back and hamstring flexibility.

Shoulders: Behind-The-Back Reach

1. In a standing position, place your left hand on the middle of your back, palm out, fingers reaching up.
2. Slide your right hand behind and down your back and try to touch your hands or fingers.
3. If they can touch you have good shoulder flexibility.
4. Switch hand positions and repeat with the other shoulder.
5. If your hands do not touch, place a ruler in the bottom hand and measure the distance between the opposing fingers.
6. If you are not within an inch of making contact, you may be susceptible to shoulder and neck pain.

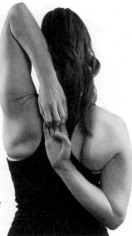

© innovatedcaptures | Thinkstock

A good indicator of shoulder flexibility is the behind-the-back reach.

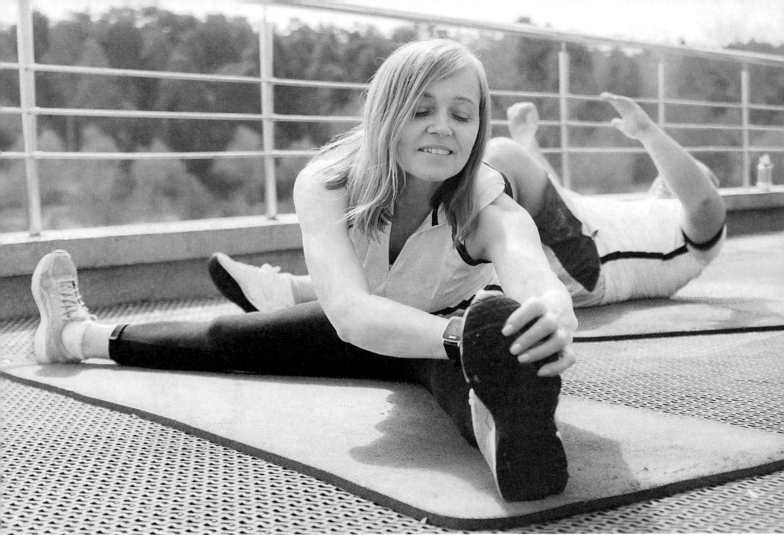

© Essik9 | Dreamstime

When stretching, remember not to bounce as it can cause injuries.

3 64 Exercises

There are two reasons for including 64 stretching and range-of-motion exercise descriptions and illustrations (plus variations) in this chapter. The first is so that you can choose which exercises are best suited to your age, physical condition, personality, and preference of styles (sitting, standing, lying, for example).

The second is to keep you from getting bored. There are, for example, three illustrated stretches just for the hamstrings, those muscles on the back of your upper legs, which are common weak areas for many older adults. If you get tired or bored doing Hamstring Lean Forward (Exercise 11), you can switch to Stairstep Hamstring Raise (Exercise 12), or Hamstring Doorway Stretch (Exercise 13). It's okay to mix things up, as long as you engage all of the areas of the body that need attention: lower body, trunk/core, and upper body.

Not Just Stretches

Flexibility exercises are not limited to stretches. Some range-of-motion movements used by patients in rehabilitation settings are safe enough to do at home. Many of the exercises described here can be modified to become range-of-motion exercises by going though the movement, but not holding a stretch position for the recommended 10 to 30 seconds. (If you have questions about which ones are appropriate, ask your physical therapist or personal trainer.)

Throughout the instructions you will see the terms "repetitions" and "sets." A repetition, or rep, is the act of performing a single stretch once. You may be asked to perform an exercise called a "Lunge" eight to 10 times. Those eight to 10 reps constitute a single "set." The instructions will suggest that you rest for a minute or two, then perform one, two, or three more "sets" of eight to 10 reps.

All of the recommended reps and sets are suggestions only. If you are beginning a flexibility training program, begin with a number with which you are comfortable, no matter how low. Then gradually build up to the suggested number of repetitions and sets to ensure that you are getting the desired effect, which is to increase your flexibility.

Bottom To Top

Finally, the stretches and exercises are arranged from bottom up—lower body to trunk/core to upper body. In most cases, the goal is to include two to three stretches for each area of the body during each workout.

The number of stretching sessions per week is up to you, but do at least two in addition to the other fitness routines—balance/mobility or core fitness or aerobic fitness, and/or strength/power—on the same day, or alternating days. (The sample programs offered in Chapter 5 follow the guideline of two to three stretches for each of the three body areas for each workout.)

All of the 64 stretches are included in the Easy Exercise Directory on page 28, which is divided into the three sections. Besides listing the exercise names, the directory lists the exercise number and page number for easy reference.

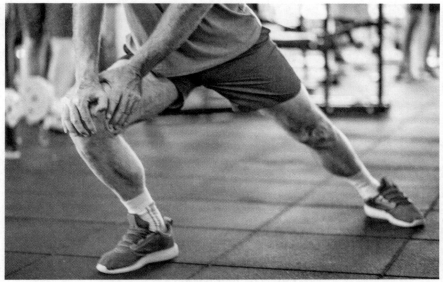
© Euroleadergroup121 | Dreamstime

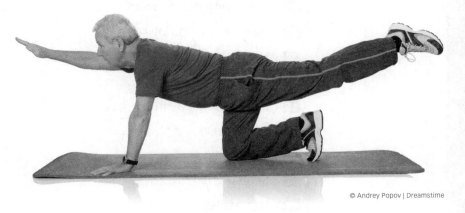
© Andrey Popov | Dreamstime

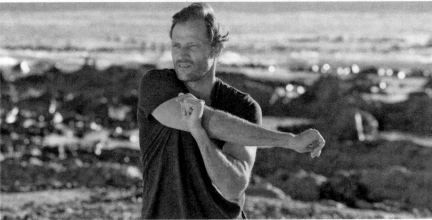
© Mimagephotography | Dreamstime

Your cool-down routine is equally as important as your warm-up routine.

Easy Exercise illustrations by Alayna Paquette

LOWER BODY FLEXIBILITY EXERCISES

TRUNK / CORE FLEXIBILITY EXERCISES

UPPER BODY FLEXIBILITY EXERCISES

TOES BACK
EXERCISE **1**

- Sit with one leg crossed over the other.
- Grasp your heel or ankle with one hand and your toes or ball of the foot in the other.
- Pull your toes up and back toward your knee/shin (don't engage your ankle) to stretch the plantar fascia tissue on the bottom of your foot.
- Hold for 10-30 seconds, relax, and repeat for a total of 2-3 reps, 1 set.
- Change positions and stretch the bottom of the opposite foot.

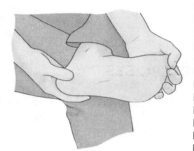

Variation #1: Complete the motion, pause for 1-3 seconds instead of holding for 10-30 seconds.

Variation #2: Sit in a sturdy chair, legs stretched out, heels on the floor. Flex your ankles so that your toes point toward you.

ANKLE FLEX/EXTEND
EXERCISE **2**

- In a sitting position, stretch your legs forward, heels on the floor.
- Flex your ankles, toes pointing up and toward your body.
- Hold for 10-30 seconds, relax, and repeat for a total of 2-3 repetitions, 1 set.
- Now flex your ankles, toes pointing down and away from your body.
- Hold for 10-30 seconds, relax, and repeat for a total of 2-3 repetitions, 1 set.

Variation: Complete the motion, pause for 1-3 seconds instead of holding for 10-30 seconds.

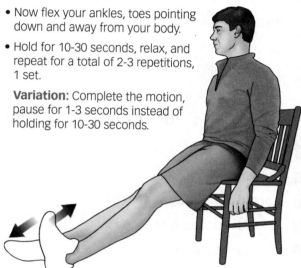

FOOT/ANKLE CIRCLES
EXERCISE **3**

- In a seated position, stretch your legs forward, heels on the floor.
- Lift one foot at a time (or both feet together) slightly off the floor and make foot and ankle circles as large as possible.
- Complete 10-20 circles, stopping halfway through to change directions.
- 1 set.

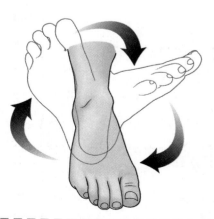

LOWER LEG
EXERCISE **4**

TOWEL STRETCH

- Sit on the floor with one or both legs extended in front.
- Wrap a towel around the bottom of one foot, holding each end of the towel in your right and left hands, respectively.
- Pull back on the towel, flexing your ankle so that the top of your foot moves toward your body. Don't bend your knee.
- Hold for 20-30 seconds, relax, and repeat for a total of 2-3 repetitions.
- 2-3 sets.
- Change positions and pull the towel back on the opposite foot.

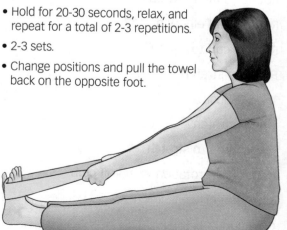

ANKLE INVERSION

- Secure one end of a resistance band to a table leg or sturdy object, and hook the other end to the inside of your forefoot.
- Keep the heel still and move your forefoot inward, pulling against the band.
- Return to the starting position to complete 1 repetition.
- Complete 5-10 reps
- After finishing your reps, switch feet and repeat.

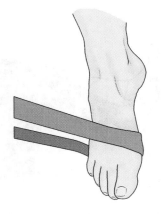

ANKLE EVERSION

- Hook the band on the outside of your forefoot, and then move your foot to the outside against the band.
- Return to the starting position to complete 1 repetition.
- Complete 5-10 reps.
- After finishing your reps, switch feet and repeat.

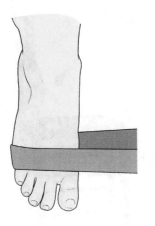

TOE RAISE/
CALF RAISE

- Stand near something to hold onto for support, such as a chair back or table, feet parallel and at shoulder width.
- Rise up on your toes to a point of resistance and hold for 10 seconds.
- Return to the starting position and repeat the movement 1-2 more times.

  Variation: Same movement, but hold for one 30-second stretch.

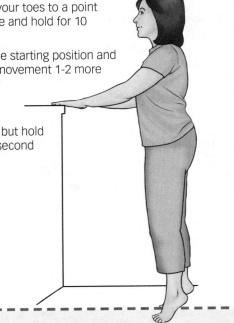

STAIRSTEP CALF RAISE

- Stand on a stair step, holding the rail for support, with the toes of both feet near the edge, heels below the stair step level, then rise on your toes.
- Hold for 10-30 seconds, then slowly return to the starting position.
- Begin with 5-6 repetitions and work up to 8-10 repetitions, 2-3 sets.

  Variation #2: Same exercise, using one foot at a time.

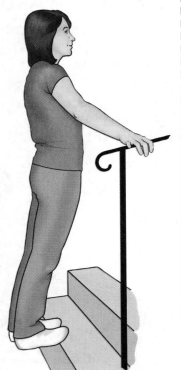

LEG CURLS

EXERCISE 9

- Stand behind a sturdy chair, holding on for balance.
- Lift your right foot and bend your leg as far as possible toward your buttocks.
- Hesitate at the top, lower your leg slowly, and repeat 8-10 times with each leg.
- 2-3 sets.
- Work toward performing the exercise without having to hold on for balance.

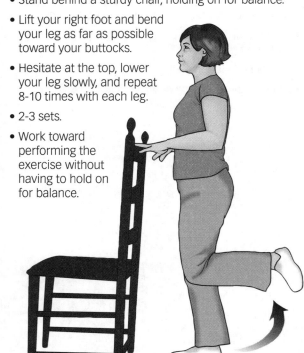

LEG EXTENSIONS

EXERCISE 10

- Sit in a sturdy straight-back chair, arms at sides, knees bent at 90 degrees
- Extend your right leg fully in front, pause, and return to the starting position.
- 8-10 reps, 2-3 sets.
- Change positions and repeat the sequence with the other leg.

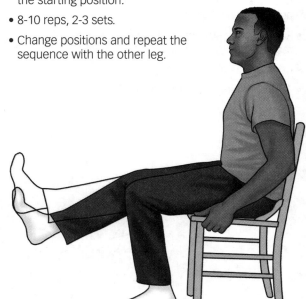

HAMSTRING LEAN FORWARD

EXERCISE 11

- Sit on the floor, legs extended forward.
- Lean forward and reach with both hands toward your toes until you feel a stretch.
- Keep your back flat and not rounded.
- Hold for 5-10 seconds, return to the starting position, and repeat 8-10 times.
- Work toward 2-3 sets.

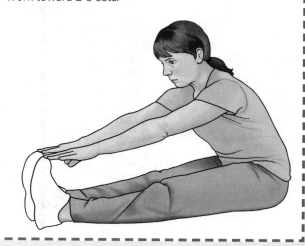

STAIRSTEP HAMSTRING RAISE

EXERCISE 12

- Stand at the bottom of the stairs, use the handrail for support, and place your left leg on the first or second step.
- Bend your right leg slightly and bend forward from the hips, keeping your back straight until you feel a stretch in the back of the thigh.
- Hold for 10-30 seconds, 2-3 sets.
- Change positions and stretch the opposite hamstring.

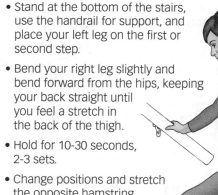
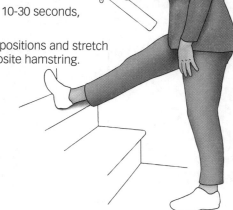

HAMSTRING DOORWAY STRETCH

EXERCISE 13

- Take a lying position in front of and slightly to the side of a doorframe.
- Extend your right leg upward and against the doorframe as far up as possible without pain or discomfort.
- Keep your left leg extended through the doorway opening.
- Hold for 20-30 seconds, 2-3 sets. Switch leg positions and repeat.

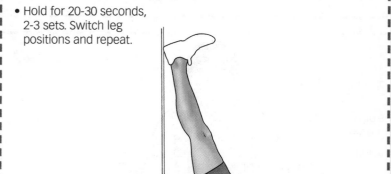

LUNGES

EXERCISE 14

- Stand with your feet hip-width apart.
- Take a long step forward (12-18 inches) with your right foot, and keep the heel of your back foot in contact with the floor. Don't extend your knee past your toes.
- Hold 1-3 seconds and return to the starting position. Repeat with the opposite foot.
- Work up to 8-10 repetitions and 2-3 sets for each leg.

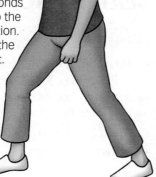

SIDE-LYING QUAD STRETCH

EXERCISE 15

- Lie on your left side, left upper arm on the floor, elbow bent, hand supporting head.
- Bend your right leg back so that the heel moves up toward your buttocks.
- At the same time, reach back and grasp your foot, pant leg, or shoe with your right hand and pull gently.
- Hold for 5-10 seconds, relax, and return to the starting position.
- 2-3 repetitions, then change positions to stretch the left quad, 2-3 sets.

PRONE QUAD

EXERCISE 16

- Lie on your stomach, left leg extended, the other bent so that your foot is above your right buttock.
- Reach back with your right hand and grasp your right foot across its top.
- Gently pull for 5-10 seconds, relax, and return to the starting position.
- Repeat 2-3 times, then change positions to stretch the opposite leg.

Variation: Perform the same exercise lying on your side.

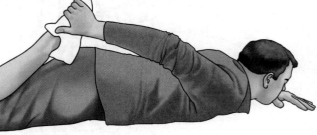

LOWER BODY FLEXIBILITY

EASY EXERCISES

SIDE LEG LIFTS

EXERCISE 17

- Lie on your left side, right leg resting on your left leg.

- Raise your right leg as high as possible without discomfort, hold for 3-5 seconds, slowly return to the starting position.

- Work up to 8-10 repetitions, 2-3 sets, with each leg.

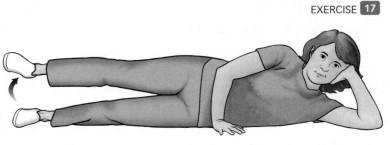

SEATED GROIN STRETCH

EXERCISE 18

- Don't use this stretch unless you have a reasonable degree of lower body flexibility.

- Sit on the floor and position your legs so the soles of your feet are touching and your knees are pointed outward to the sides.

- Place your elbows or forearms against your knees and gently press down.

- Hold for 3-5 seconds and return to the starting position.

- Gradually increase the number of repetitions to 8-10, 2-3 sets.

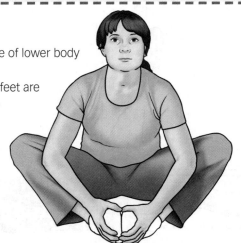

LEG SWINGS

EXERCISE 19

- Holding onto a chair for support, stand on one leg and swing the other, using the hip joint to move your leg in a front to back motion.

- Maintain a pendulum-like motion, but limit the distance off the ground to no more than 12 inches.

- 10-20 swings for each leg, 1-2 sets

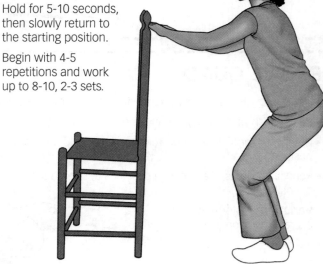

MODIFIED SQUATS

EXERCISE 20

- Stand behind a sturdy chair or at arm's length from a counter top, feet comfortably apart, hands on the top of a chair or counter.

- Slowly lower your hips and knees to assume a semi-squat position, but not low enough so that your upper legs are parallel to the floor.

- Hold for 5-10 seconds, then slowly return to the starting position.

- Begin with 4-5 repetitions and work up to 8-10, 2-3 sets.

HAMSTRING STRETCH WITH TOWEL

- Lie on your back, and place a towel, strap, or belt over the ball of your raised foot.
- Gently pull the strap and lift your leg toward your head until you reach a point of resistance. Bend your knee if needed.
- Point your toes upward and hold for 10-30 seconds.
- Change positions and repeat the movement with the opposite leg to complete 1 set, 2-3 sets.

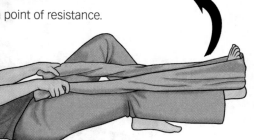

RESISTANCE BAND CLAMSHELLS

- Lie on your left side, right leg on top of the left, knees comfortably bent.
- With a resistance band wrapped around your knees, rotate the right leg up until your leg makes a 90-degree angle to the floor.
- Hold for 1-2 seconds and slowly return to the starting position.
- Change positions and complete the same number of repetitions and sets with the opposite leg, 2-3 sets.

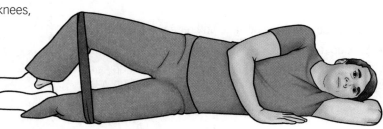

STABILITY BALL WALL SQUATS

- In a standing position, place a stability ball behind your back against a wall at waist level with your hands to your sides.
- Slowly bend your knees into a squat position, upper legs parallel to the floor, allowing the ball to roll up your back.
- Hold for 2-3 seconds, straighten your legs, and slowly return to the starting position.
- 3-5 reps, 2-3 sets.

  Variation: Bend your knees and lower your body to a semi-squat position.

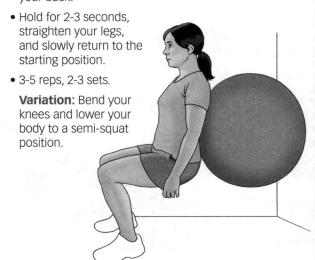

ACHILLES WALL STRETCH

- From a standing position facing a wall with one foot forward, arm's length from the wall, lean forward and place both hands on the wall.
- Keep both feet flat on the surface as you lean forward.
- Hold for 20-30 seconds, return to the starting position, and repeat for a total of 2-3 times.
- Change positions and stretch the Achilles tendon of the opposite foot.

  Variation: Begin with both feet even, hands on the wall, and lean forward as if doing a wall push-up, keeping both feet flat on the floor.

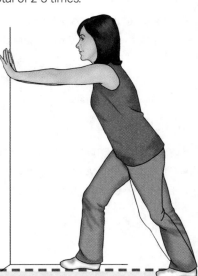

BACK EXTENSION #1

EXERCISE 25

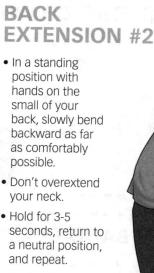

- Lie face down, hands flat on floor, slightly forward as if beginning a push up.
- Slowly push up and relax your back into an arched position.
- Hold for 3-5 seconds.
- Return to the starting position and repeat 8-10 times.
- Work up to 2-3 sets.

   Variation: Instead of extending your arms as if doing a push-up, let the weight of your upper body rest on your elbows.

BACK EXTENSION #2

EXERCISE 26

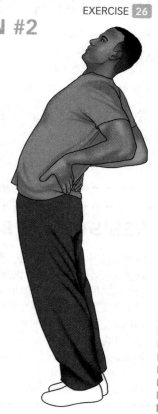

- In a standing position with hands on the small of your back, slowly bend backward as far as comfortably possible.
- Don't overextend your neck.
- Hold for 3-5 seconds, return to a neutral position, and repeat.
- Begin with 5-6 extensions and work up to 8-10 repetitions, 2-3 sets, resting between sets.

BACK EXTENSION #3

EXERCISE 27

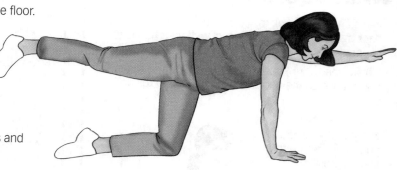

- Begin from a hands and knees position on the floor.
- Carefully lift then extend your left arm and right leg at the same time.
- Hold for 2-3 seconds to complete 1 rep.
- Repeat the motion with right arm and left leg extended.
- Work up to 8-10 reps, 2-3 sets

   Variation: Lift, rather than extend, your arms and legs.

TRUNK LIFTS

EXERCISE 28

- Lie on your stomach, hands behind your head.
- Without arching your back, slowly lift your head and shoulders slightly off the floor.
- Hold for 5 seconds, then return to the starting position.
- Repeat 4-5 times, 2-3 sets.

TORSO STRETCH

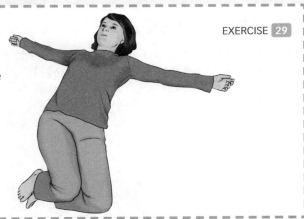

- Lie on your back, legs bent, feet flat on the floor.
- Keeping your knees together, roll your legs to the left toward the floor until you feel the stretch.
- Keep your shoulders grounded.
- Hold for 5-10 seconds and slowly return to the starting position. Repeat to the right side to complete 1 rep.
- Work up to 8-10 repetitions, 2-3 sets.

TORSO ROTATION

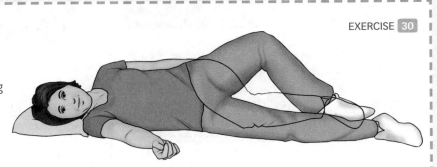

- Lie on your right side, right leg slightly bent.
- Place your left foot behind your right leg and then rotate your knee to the floor.
- Hold for 5-10 seconds and work up to 8-10 repetitions on each side, 2-3 sets.

STANDING SIDE BENDS

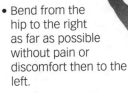

- Stand shoulder-width apart, extend your arms upward and clasp your hands, palms in.
- Bend from the hip to the right as far as possible without pain or discomfort then to the left.
- Hold each bend for 5-10 seconds and repeat 8-10 times on each side, 2-3 sets.

Variation: Same movement, but place one hand on your hip, the other up in the air.

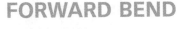

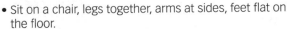

FORWARD BEND

- Sit on a chair, legs together, arms at sides, feet flat on the floor.
- Lean/bend forward, bringing your shoulders down toward your knees as far as comfortably possible.
- Keep your back flat and not rounded.
- Hold for 5-10 seconds, slowly return to the starting position, and repeat 1-2 times to complete a set.
- 2-3 sets.

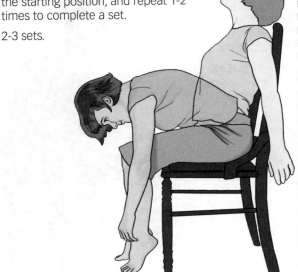
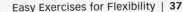

KNEES TO CHEST

EXERCISE 33

- Lie on your back, wrap your hands around your bent left leg below the knee, and slowly pull the knee toward your chest.
- Hold for 10-30 seconds and repeat 2-3 times.
- Change positions and pull the right knee toward your chest.
- 2-3 sets.

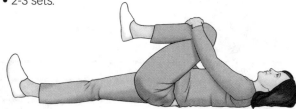

Variation #1: Assume the same position, but bring both knees up at the same time.

Variation #2: Sit in a straight chair and bring up one knee at a time toward your chest.

Variation #3: In a standing position, bring up one knee at a time toward your chest. (Stand with your back to a wall for support, if needed.)

SEATED HIP STRETCH

EXERCISE 35

- Sit in a straight-back chair, right leg crossed over and resting on the left leg.
- Gently press down on your right knee with your right hand and lean forward slightly.
- Hold for 10-30 seconds, relax, and return to the starting position.
- Work up to 8-10 repetitions, then change positions with the left leg crossed over your right leg.
- 2-3 sets.

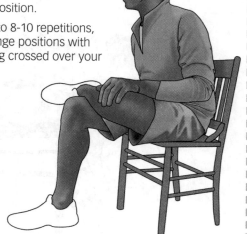

BRIDGES

EXERCISE 34

- Lie on your back, feet flat on the floor, arms extended and at your sides.
- Slowly raise your hips off the floor as high as possible without arching your spine.
- Hold for 2-3 seconds, 8-10 reps, 2-3 sets.

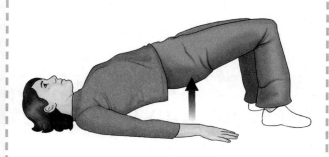

FULL BODY STRETCH #1

EXERCISE 36

- Stand with feet shoulder-width apart.
- Keep your feet grounded and raise both arms up and over your head until you feel a stretch.
- Hold for 3-5 seconds and repeat 5-6 times.
- Work up to 8-10 reps, 2-3 sets.

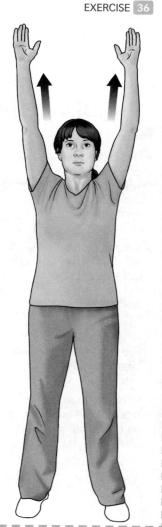

FULL BODY STRETCH #2

EXERCISE 37

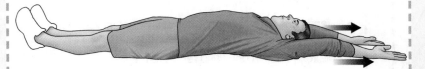

- Lie on your back, legs extended, arms extended above your head.
- Try to make your body longer by stretching your legs and feet as far as they can reach in one direction while stretching your arms and hands as far as they can reach in the opposite direction.
- Hold for 3-5 seconds, relax, and repeat 5-6 times.
- 1 set only at first then increase to 2-3 sets.

LOWER TRUNK ROTATION

EXERCISE 39

- Lie on your back, knees bent, hands behind your head.
- Keep your shoulders flat on the floor and roll your knees to one side, touching or almost touching the floor.
- Hold for 3-5 seconds, then roll your knees back to the original position.
- Roll your knees to the opposite side and back to complete 1 rep.
- Work up to 8-10 repetitions, 2-3 sets.

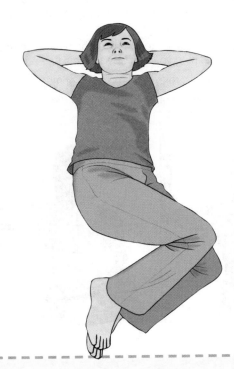

SEATED TWISTS

EXERCISE 38

- Sit up straight in a chair, arms crossed over your chest or placed down alongside your body.
- Rotate your shoulders as far in one direction as possible without discomfort.
- Hold for 3-5 seconds, return to the starting position, and repeat to the other side to complete 1 rep.
- Work up to 8-10 reps, 2-3 sets.

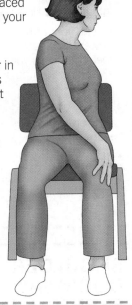

STANDING TWISTS

EXERCISE 40

- In a standing position, hold a golf club, broom handle, or similar with both hands behind your back at waist level.
- Rotate your shoulders first to the right as far as comfortably possible then to the left.
- Hold each right side/ left side position for 3-5 seconds, relax, and repeat 8-10 times, 2-3 sets.

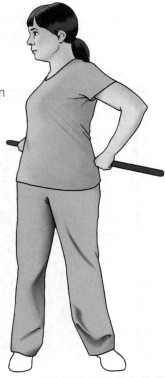

OVERHEAD REACH

EXERCISE 41

- Sitting or standing, arms up and over your head with fingers interlocked, palms up.
- Extend your arms upward until you feel a stretch in your shoulders and upper back.
- Hold for 10-30 seconds and return to the starting position.
- 8-10 reps, 2-3 sets.

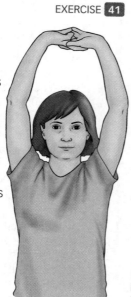

FORWARD REACH

EXERCISE 42

- Arms forward in front of you, palms in or out.
- Extend your arms forward and slightly up until you feel a stretch in your shoulders and upper back.
- Hold for 10-30 seconds and return to the starting position.
- 8-10 repetitions, 2-3 sets.

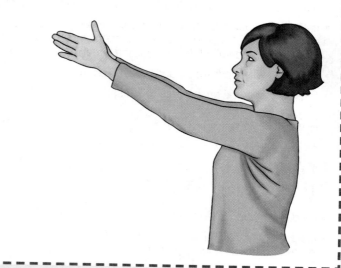

SHOULDER DOORWAY STRETCH #1

EXERCISE 43

- Stand in front of an open doorway, feet staggered, arms raised so that upper arms are parallel to the floor.
- Place your palms against the sides of the doorframe and lean forward.
- Hold for 20-30 seconds, relax, and repeat 1-3 times.
- 2-3 sets.

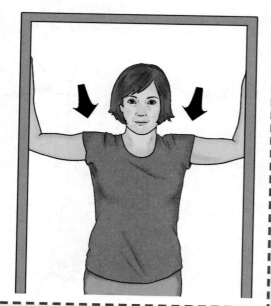

SHOULDER DOORWAY STRETCH #2

EXERCISE 44

- Stand near the side of a doorway, feet staggered, left arm up and bent at 90 degrees, palm against doorframe above head level.
- Slowly turn your upper body to the right and away from the doorframe while keeping your left arm in the same position.
- Hold for 20-30 seconds, relax, and repeat 1-2 times.
- Change positions and repeat the stretch with the opposite arm against the doorframe.

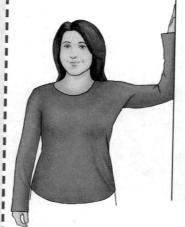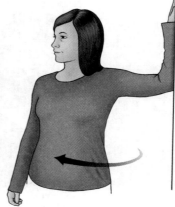

SHOULDER SQUEEZE

EXERCISE 45

- Stand or sit with elbows bent at your sides.
- Push back with your elbows and squeeze your shoulder blades together.
- Hold for 10-30 seconds, relax, 2-3 repetitions.
- 2-3 sets.

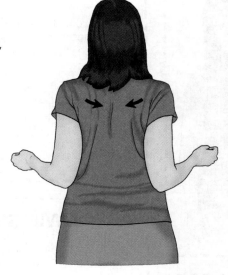

SHOULDER ROLL

EXERCISE 46

- Standing position, arms down and at sides.
- Gently roll your shoulders back and down, trying to make your shoulder blades touch with each roll.
- 5-10 rotations, 2-3 sets.

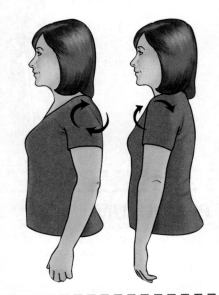

ARM CIRCLES

EXERCISE 47

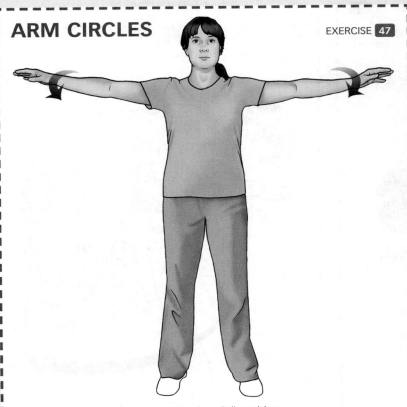

- Hold both arms out to your sides in a "T" position.
- Make 10-20 slow counter-clockwise circles with your arms.
- Stop, relax, and repeat the movement 10-12 times in the opposite direction.

HEAD TURN

EXERCISE 48

- Sit or stand, slowly turning your head to the right until you feel a stretch, but without straining.
- Hold for 10-30 seconds, rest, 3-5 reps, 2 sets.
- Repeat the motion to the left side, 3-5 reps, 2-3 sets

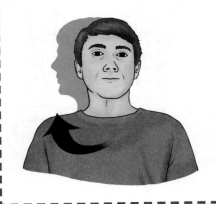

NECK TILT

EXERCISE **49**

- Sit or stand, slowly tilting your head to the left and toward your shoulder as far as comfortably possible.
- Hold for 10-30 seconds, 3-5 reps, 2 sets.
- Repeat the motion tilting your head to the right, 3-5 reps, 2 sets.

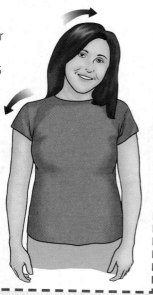

CHIN TUCK

EXERCISE **50**

- Standing or seated, head up, looking straight ahead.
- Lower your chin toward your chest until you feel a stretch in the back of your neck.
- Hold for 10-30 seconds, 3-5 reps, 2 sets.

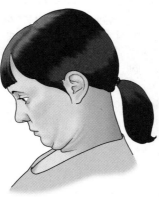

PENDULUM

EXERCISE **51**

- Stand and bend at the waist, one arm hanging down like a pendulum, the other holding onto a chair back or table for support.
- Rotate your hanging arm in a clockwise circle 10-20 times. Repeat in the opposite direction.
- Switch arm positions and repeat.

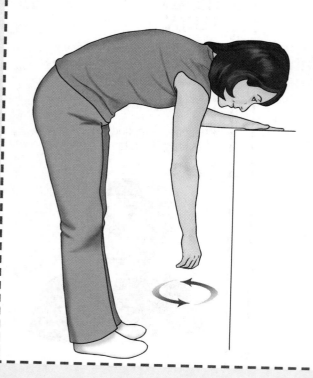

ARM SWINGS

EXERCISE **52**

- Begin in the pendulum position, bent at the waist, one arm hanging down.
- Move your hanging arm as far back as it will go without pain, then swing it forward in the opposite direction.
- Repeat the motion with the other arm.
- 10-20 reps for each arm.

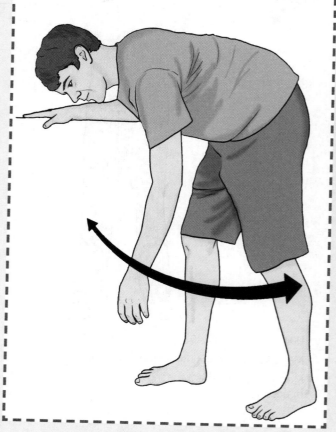

WALL WALK

- Place one hand on a wall at shoulder height.
- Walk your fingers up the wall as far as comfortably possible.
- When you reach the highest point, hold for 10 seconds, lower your arms, relax, and repeat twice, trying to walk your fingers higher each time.
- Switch arms and repeat; 2-3 sets.

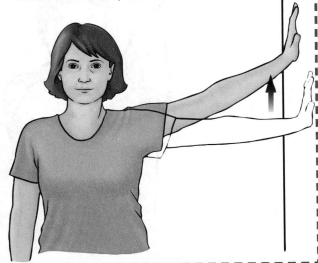

ROTATOR CUFF ELBOW PULL #1

- Stand or sit and position one arm so that it crosses your chest.
- Grasp your elbow with the opposite hand and pull it across the front of your body.
- Hold for 3-5 seconds, relax, and repeat 8-10 times, 2-3 sets with each arm.

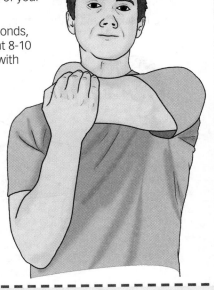

ROTATOR CUFF ELBOW PULL #2

- Stand or sit and position your right elbow next to your head, arm bent, hand between your shoulder blades.
- Use your left hand to pull the right elbow slightly and gently to the left. (Note: It won't go far.)
- Hold for 3-5 seconds, relax, and repeat 8-10 times, 2-3 sets with each arm.

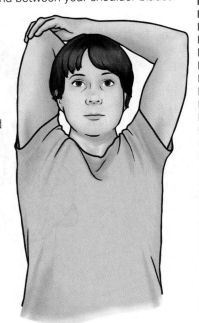

ROTATOR CUFF TOWEL PULL

- Stand or sit and hold one end of a towel in your right hand, behind your head.
- Grasp the other end of the towel (hanging down) with the other hand.
- Pull up gently with your right hand until you feel tension and hold for 3-10 seconds; repeat once or twice, and change arm positions,
- 2 sets of 1 or 2 pulls.

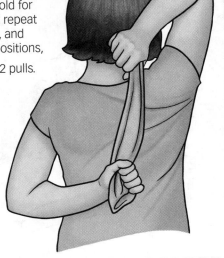

FOREARM STRETCH EXERCISE 57

- Sit or stand, extending your left arm forward, parallel to the floor, palm forward.
- Extend your right arm to grasp the fingers of the left hand.
- Gently pull back your fingertips toward your shoulders.
- Hold for 10-30 seconds, rest, and repeat.
- Change positions and stretch the opposite forearm.

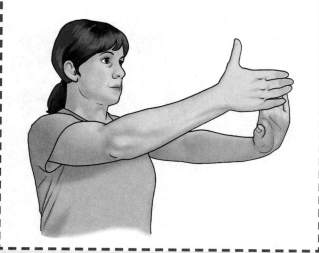

TRICEPS PUSH EXERCISE 58

- Stand or sit, right hand on right shoulder.
- Use your left hand to grasp your right elbow, pushing it upward toward the ceiling until you feel a stretch in the triceps (the muscles under your upper arm).
- Hold 5-10 seconds, relax, and repeat once.
- 1-2 sets for each arm.

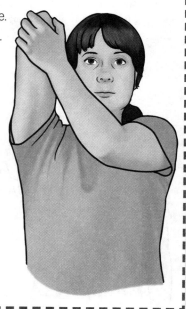

FINGER STRETCH EXERCISE 59

- Use the palm of your right hand to gently pull the fingers of the left hand, bending them back slightly.
- Hold for 3-5 seconds, relax, and repeat 5-6 times.
- Change positions and stretch the fingers of the opposite hand.

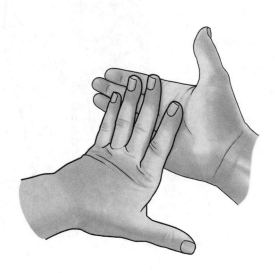

WRIST/FOREARM STRETCH EXERCISE 60

- Right arm, hand, and fingers extended.
- Use your left hand to gently pull the right fingers until you feel a stretch in the wrist.
- Hold for 20-30 seconds, then bend your right wrist downward, using your left hand to gently assist the stretch in the opposite direction.
- 2-3 reps for each wrist.

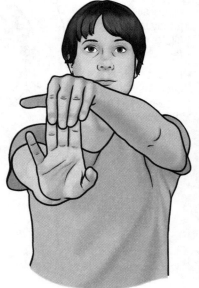

UPPER BODY ROTATION WITH GOLF CLUB

EXERCISE 61

- Sit or stand, holding a golf club (or broom handle) with hands at shoulder width, arms extended.
- Rotate the club (and your upper body) to the right as far as possible without straining, and then to the left.
- Hold for 1-2 seconds on each side and repeat to each side 8-10 times.
- 1-2 sets.

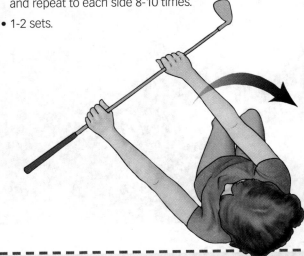

SNOW ANGELS

EXERCISE 62

- Lie on your back with your knees bent and feet flat on the floor.
- Extend your arms out at a 45-degree angle.
- Slowly move through a "snow angel" motion by sliding your hands up toward your head, while your arms stay in contact with the floor, until you reach the full extension without any pain or discomfort.
- Avoid arching your low back or shrugging your shoulders.
- If it is too difficult at first, bend your elbows.
- Repeat the movement 15-20 times.

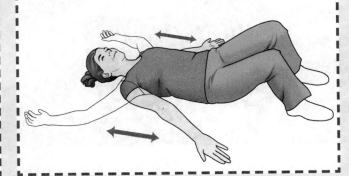

COW CURL

EXERCISE 63

- Sit up straight on the front edge of a chair with your feet on the floor. Inhale.
- On the exhale, slowly curl your spine, drawing the middle of the upper back toward the back of the chair.
- Expand your chest and look up. Hold for 5 seconds and then return to starting position.
- Repeat 3-5 times, 2-3 sets.

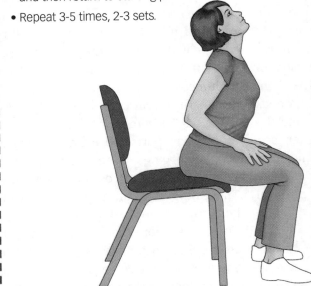

CAT CURL

EXERCISE 64

- Sit up straight on the center of a chair with your feet on the floor. Inhale.
- On the exhale, round your spine toward the ceiling, making sure to keep your shoulders and knees in position. Extend your arms.
- Release your head toward the floor, but don't force your chin to your chest.
- Hold for 5 seconds and then return to starting position.
- Repeat 3-5 times, 2-3 sets.

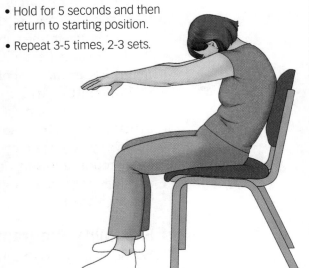

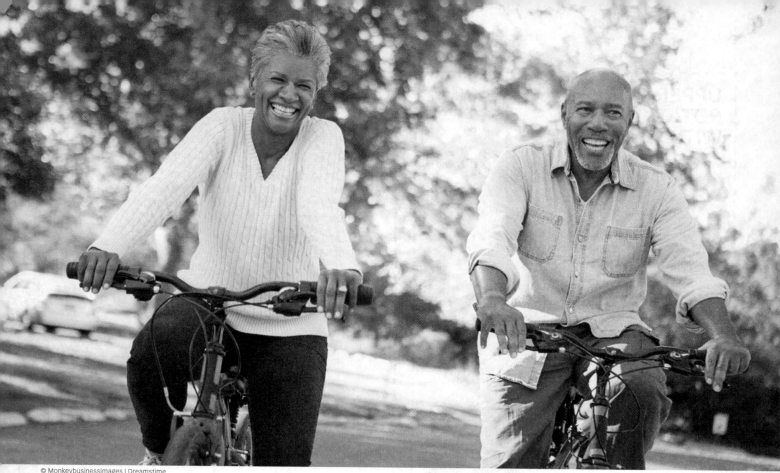
© Monkeybusinessimages | Dreamstime

Cardio exercises such as bike riding are a great way to maintain flexibility.

4 21 Exercise Packages

Use your choice of the 64 stretching and range-of-motion, exercises in Chapter 3 to design your own program, or follow the sample routines that follow.

Flexibility Exercise Finder

The Flexibility Exercise Finder lets you quickly scan the names of all the exercises and programs in the report, plus the pages where they are found. If you are looking for flexibility exercises for tennis, for example, look for the "Tennis" title in the center column, check the page number on the right, and flip to that page for tennis-specific exercises. This way you can put together mini flexibility routines to support your favorite activities or to address specific physical issues or needs.

Flexibility Programs

The flexibility programs include a five- to 10-minute dynamic stretching warm up, which should be challenging enough to break a sweat and increase circulation. Brisk walking, light calisthenics, treadmills, elliptical, and stationary bikes are typical warm-up activities. A cool-down period won't hurt, but is not as necessary if you are doing only flexibility exercises.

However, a proper cool down is required if you follow your flexibility routine with aerobic fitness, strength, or other fitness components, which helps with recovery and reduces soreness.

The first section, Activity-Specific Exercises & Stretches, includes routines for popular sports and activities, such as walking/jogging, swimming, cycling, golf, tennis, skiing, and post-gym workouts. These programs can help increase your performance and reduce risk of injury. The next section, Special Situation Exercises & Stretches, are those to consider if you are an exercise beginner, "weekend warrior," or stuck in certain long-duration activities, like watching television, sitting at a desk or computer, or traveling in a car or plane. You can do them as preparation for these activities or afterward.

The section also highlights stretching routines to offer relief to common hot spots like a stiff back or neck, achy knees, and sore feet, as well as programs focused on improving the flexibility and conditioning of your major joints: neck, shoulders, hips, knees, and feet and ankles. (Note: You can modify each exercise routine according to your specific physical condition. Make sure to consult with your doctor before beginning any new exercise program.)

FLEXIBILITY EXERCISE FINDER	PAGE
ACTIVITY-SPECIFIC EXERCISES & STRETCHES	
Walking/Hiking	48
Swimming	48
Skiing	48
Tennis	48
Jogging	49
Golf	49
Cycling	49
Beginning an Exercise Program	50
Post-Gym Workouts	50
Weekend Warriors	50
Watching TV	51
In A Car/On A Plane	51
Sitting At A Desk/Computer	51
SPECIAL SITUATION EXERCISES & STRETCHES	
Sore Back	52
Stiff Knees	52
Tight Neck/Shoulders	52
Neck	53
Shoulders	53
Hips	53
Knees	53
Feet/Ankles	53

WALKING/HIKING

☑ **Warm-up**

☑ **ANKLE FLEX/EXTEND**
- Exercise: `2`
- Reps: 1 for 10-30 seconds
- Sets: 2-3

☑ **FOOT/ANKLE CIRCLES**
- Exercise: `3`
- Reps: 10-20 circles for each foot
- Sets: 1

☑ **LEG CURLS**
- Exercise: `9`
- Reps: 10-15 times with each leg
- Sets: 2-3

☑ **LEG SWINGS**
- Exercise: `19`
- Reps: 10-20 for each leg
- Sets: 1

SWIMMING

☑ **Warm-up**

☑ **BACK EXTENSION #1**
- Exercise: `25`
- Reps: 8-10
- Sets: 2-3

☑ **OVERHEAD REACH**
- Exercise: `41`
- Reps: 8-10
- Sets: 2

☑ **FORWARD REACH**
- Exercise: `42`
- Reps: 8-10
- Sets: 2-3

☑ **TRICEPS PUSH**
- Exercise: `58`
- Reps: 1-2 for each arm
- Sets: 1-2

SKIING

☑ **Warm-up**

☑ **LUNGES**
- Exercise: `14`
- Reps: 8-10
- Sets: 2-3

☑ **SEATED GROIN STRETCH**
- Exercise: `18`
- Reps: 8-10
- Sets: 2-3

☑ **MODIFIED SQUATS**
- Exercise: `20`
- Reps: Begin with 4-5, work up to 8-10
- Sets: 2-3

☑ **FORWARD REACH**
- Exercise: `42`
- Reps: 8-10
- Sets: 2-3

TENNIS

☑ **Warm-up**

☑ **ACHILLES WALL STRETCH**
- Exercise: `24`
- Reps: 2-3
- Sets: 1-2

☑ **LEG CURLS**
- Exercise: `9`
- Reps: 10-15 times with each leg
- Sets: 2-3

☑ **STANDING SIDE BENDS**
- Exercise: `31`
- Reps: 8-10
- Sets: 2-3

☑ **OVERHEAD REACH**
- Exercise: `41`
- Reps: 8-10
- Sets: 2

JOGGING

☑ **Warm-up**

☑ **LEG CURLS**
  - Exercise: 9
  - Reps: 10-15 times with each leg
  - 2-3 sets

☑ **LEG EXTENSIONS**
  - Exercise: 10
  - Reps: 8-10
  - Sets: 2-3

☑ **LUNGES**
  - Exercise: 14
  - Reps: 8-10
  - Sets: 2-3

☑ **LEG SWINGS**
  - Exercise: 19
  - Reps: 10-20 for each leg
  - Sets: 1

☑ **STANDING SIDE BENDS**
  - Exercise: 31
  - Reps: 8-10
  - Sets: 2-3

GOLF

☑ **Warm-up**

☑ **ACHILLES WALL STRETCH**
  - Exercise: 24
  - Reps: 2-3
  - Sets: 2-3

☑ **BACK EXTENSION #2**
  - Exercise: 26
  - Reps: 8-10
  - Sets: 2-3

☑ **STANDING SIDE BENDS**
  - Exercise: 31
  - Reps: 8-10
  - Sets: 2-3

☑ **FULL BODY STRETCH #1**
  - Exercise: 36
  - Reps: 8-10
  - Sets: 2-3

☑ **UPPER BODY ROTATION WITH GOLF CLUB**
  - Exercise: 61
  - Reps: 8-10
  - Sets: 2-3

CYCLING

☑ **Warm-up**

☑ **LEG CURLS**
  - Exercise: 9
  - Reps: 8-10
  - Sets: 2-3

☑ **LEG EXTENSIONS**
  - Exercise: 10
  - Reps: 8-10
  - Sets: 2-3

☑ **HAMSTRING LEAN FORWARD**
  - Exercise: 11
  - Reps: 8-10
  - Sets: 2-3

☑ **MODIFIED SQUATS**
  - Exercise: 20
  - Reps: Begin with 4-5, work up to 8-10
  - Sets: 2-3

☑ **FORWARD BEND**
  - Exercise: 32
  - Reps: 2-3
  - Sets: 2-3

BEGINNING AN EXERCISE PROGRAM

☑ **Warm-up**

☑ **ACHILLES WALL STRETCH**
- Exercise: 24
- Reps: 2-3
- Sets: 1-2

☑ **LUNGES**
- Exercise: 14
- Reps: 5-6, work up to 8-10
- Sets: 1-2, work up to 2-3

☑ **KNEES TO CHEST**
- Exercise: 33
- Reps: 5-6, work up to 8-10
- Sets: 1-2, work up to 2-3

☑ **OVERHEAD REACH**
- Exercise: 41
- Reps: 5-6, work up to 8-10
- Sets: 1-2, work up to 2-3

POST-GYM WORKOUTS

☑ **SEATED GROIN STRETCH**
- Exercise: 18
- Reps: 5-6
- Sets: 1-2

☑ **BACK EXTENSION #2**
- Exercise: 26
- Reps: 5-6
- Sets: 1-2

☑ **ROTATOR CUFF ELBOW PULL #1**
- Exercise: 54
- Reps: 5-6
- Sets: 1-2

☑ **ROTATOR CUFF ELBOW PULL #2**
- Exercise: 55
- Reps: 8-10
- Sets: 2-3

WEEKEND WARRIORS

☑ **LOWER LEG TOWEL STRETCH**
- Exercise: 4
- Reps: 2-3
- Sets: 2-3

☑ **TOE RAISE/CALF RAISE**
- Exercise: 7
- Reps: 8-10
- Sets: 2-3

☑ **LUNGES**
- Exercise: 14
- Reps: 8-10
- Sets: 2-3

☑ **TORSO STRETCH**
- Exercise: 29
- Reps: 8-10
- Sets: 2-3

☑ **SHOULDER DOORWAY STRETCH #1**
- Exercise: 43
- Reps: 5-6
- Sets: 2-3

☑ **OVERHEAD REACH**
- Exercise: 41
- Reps: 5-6, work up to 8-10
- Sets: 1-2, work up to 2-3

WATCHING TV

☑ **ANKLE FLEX/EXTEND**
- Exercise: `2`
- Reps: 2-3
- Sets: 2-3

☑ **SEATED GROIN**
- Exercise: `18`
- Reps: 8-10
- Sets: 2-3

☑ **SEATED TWISTS**
- Exercise: `38`
- Reps: 8-10
- Sets: 2-3

☑ **FORWARD BEND**
- Exercise: `32`
- Reps: 1-3
- Sets: 2-3

☑ **OVERHEAD REACH**
- Exercise: `41`
- Reps: 5-6, work up to 8-10
- Sets: 1-2, work up to 2-3

☑ **SHOULDER SQUEEZE**
- Exercise: `45`
- Reps: 2-3
- Sets: 2-3

IN A CAR/ON A PLANE

☑ **ANKLE FLEX/EXTEND**
- Exercise: `2`
- Reps: 1 for 10-30 seconds
- Sets: 2-3

☑ **FOOT/ANKLE CIRCLES**
- Exercise: `3`
- Reps: 10-20 circles for each foot
- Sets: 1

☑ **KNEES TO CHEST, VARIATION #2**
- Exercise: `33`
- Reps: 2-3
- Sets: 2-3

☑ **OVERHEAD REACH**
- Exercise: `41`
- Reps: 5-6, work up to 8-10
- Sets: 1-2, work up to 2-3

☑ **SHOULDER ROLL**
- Exercise: `46`
- Reps: 5-10
- Sets: 2-3

☑ **HEAD TURN**
- Exercise: `48`
- Reps: 3
- Sets: 2-3

SITTING AT A DESK OR COMPUTER

☑ **KNEES TO CHEST, VARIATION #2**
- Exercise: `33`
- Reps: 2-3
- Sets: 2-3

☑ **OVERHEAD REACH**
- Exercise: `41`
- Reps: 5-6, work up to 8-10
- Sets: 1-2, work up to 2-3

☑ **SHOULDER SQUEEZE**
- Exercise: `45`
- Reps: 2-3
- Sets: 2-3

☑ **SHOULDER ROLL**
- Exercise: `46`
- Reps: 5-10
- Sets: 2-3

☑ **HEAD TURN**
- Exercise: `48`
- Reps: 3-5
- Sets: 2-3

☑ **NECK TILT**
- Exercise: `49`
- Reps: 5-10
- Sets: 2-3

Note: Modify each exercise according to physical condition.

SORE BACK

☑ **BACK EXTENSION #1**
- Exercise: 25
- Reps: 8-10
- Sets: 2-3

☑ **BACK EXTENSION #3**
- Exercise: 27
- Reps: 5-6, work up to 8-10
- Sets: 2-3

☑ **KNEES TO CHEST**
- Exercise: 33
- Reps: 2-3
- Sets: 2-3

☑ **FULL BODY STRETCH #1**
- Exercise: 36
- Reps: 5-6, work up to 8-10
- Sets: 2-3

STIFF KNEES

☑ **LEG CURLS**
- Exercise: 9
- Reps: 8-10
- Sets: 2-3

☑ **LEG EXTENSIONS**
- Exercise: 10
- Reps: 8-10
- Sets: 2-3

☑ **LUNGES**
- Exercise: 14
- Reps: 8-10
- Sets: 2-3

☑ **MODIFIED SQUATS**
- Exercise: 20
- Reps: Begin with 4-5, work up to 8-10
- Sets: 2-3

☑ **KNEES TO CHEST, VARIATION #2**
- Exercise: 33
- Reps: 2-3
- Sets: 2-3

TIGHT NECK/SHOULDERS

☑ **OVERHEAD REACH**
- Exercise: 41
- Reps: 5-6, work up to 8-10
- Sets: 1-2, work up to 2-3

☑ **SHOULDER DOORWAY STRETCH #1**
- Exercise: 43
- Reps: 1-3
- Sets: 2-3

☑ **SHOULDER SQUEEZE**
- Exercise: 45
- Reps: 2-3
- Sets: 2-3

☑ **SHOULDER ROLL**
- Exercise: 46
- Reps: 5-10
- Sets: 2-3

☑ **HEAD TURN**
- Exercise: 48
- Reps: 3-5
- Sets: 2-3

☑ **ROTATOR CUFF ELBOW PULL #1**
- Exercise: 54
- Reps: 8-10
- Sets: 2-3

NECK

☑ **HEAD TURN**
- Exercise: `48`
- Reps: 3-5
- Sets: 2-3

☑ **NECK TILT**
- Exercise: `49`
- Reps: 3-5
- Sets: 2-3

☑ **CHIN TUCK**
- Exercise: `50`
- Reps: 3-5
- Sets: 2-3

SHOULDERS

☑ **PENDULUM**
- Exercise: `51`
- Reps: 10-20 circles in each direction
- Sets: 1-2

☑ **ARM SWINGS**
- Exercise: `52`
- Reps: 10-20 for each arm
- Sets: 1-2

☑ **WALL WALK**
- Exercise: `53`
- Reps: 2-3
- Sets: 1-2

HIPS

☑ **SIDE LEG LIFTS**
- Exercise: `17`
- Reps: 3-5
- Sets: 1-2

☑ **LEG SWINGS**
- Exercise: `19`
- Reps: 3-5
- Sets: 1-2

☑ **SEATED HIP STRETCH**
- Exercise: `35`
- Reps: 8-10
- Sets: 2-3

KNEES

☑ **LEG CURLS**
- Exercise: `9`
- Reps: 8-10
- Sets: 2-3

☑ **LEG EXTENSIONS**
- Exercise: `10`
- Reps: 8-10
- Sets: 2-3

FEET/ANKLES

☑ **TOES BACK, VARIATION #1**
- Exercise: `1`
- Reps: 2-3
- Sets: 1

☑ **ANKLE FLEX/EXTEND**
- Exercise: `2`
- Reps: 2-3
- Sets: 1

☑ **FOOT/ANKLE CIRCLES**
- Exercise: `3`
- Reps: 10-20 circles
- Sets: 1

SPECIAL SITUATION EXERCISES & STRETCHES

EASY EXERCISES

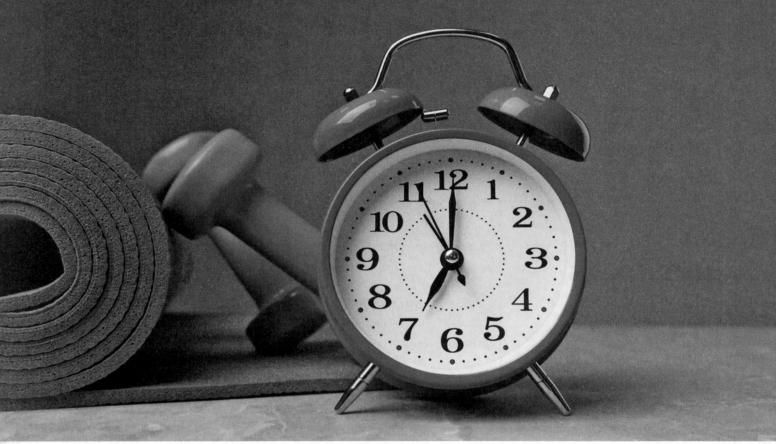

Keeping track of your routine can be pivotal to your progress.

5 The Workbook

People who engage in a successful fitness program, including a flexibility component, do three things: schedule it, do the exercises, and keep a record of it. On the pages that follow are tools to help you accomplish all three.

Daily Flexibility Log

The first tool is a Daily Flexibility Log which helps you schedule and track your progress. Makes copies of it and check off the exercises, number of repetitions, and number of sets on a daily and ongoing basis. Seeing a record of your progress and what you have accomplished is a proven method of adhering to a program.

Eight-Week Flexibility Workout

The Eight-Week Flexibility Workout (see pages 56-59) outlines weekly flexibility workouts that cover your upper body, trunk/core, and lower body. You can either perform these routines on alternating days from your regular exercise, or add them to the end of your workouts.

Following this schedule can help you become familiar with various types of stretches and establish a routine. At the end of the eight-week period, you can begin again, or use these programs as a template to create your own routines.

There is a different stretching program for each week. However, these are only suggestions, so feel free to switch out individual stretches, but make sure they address the corresponding body area. For example, replace an upper body stretch with one from the same category. If you find a weekly program you enjoy, you can repeat it.

Flexibility is essential to staying active, mobile, and independent, and requires the same attention and dedication as any other aspect of your health. You will find that when your flexibility improves, your overall wellness will follow.

DAILY FLEXIBILITY LOG

DAY	EXERCISE NAME	NUMBER	REPS	SETS	NOTES
MONDAY	(EXAMPLE) Seated Twists	19	10	2	
MONDAY					
MONDAY					
TUESDAY					
TUESDAY					
TUESDAY					
WEDNESDAY					
WEDNESDAY					
WEDNESDAY					
THURSDAY					
THURSDAY					
THURSDAY					
FRIDAY					
FRIDAY					
FRIDAY					
SATURDAY					
SATURDAY					
SATURDAY					
SUNDAY					
SUNDAY					
SUNDAY					

PROGRAM: WEEK #1

☑ **LOWER LEG TOWEL STRETCH**
- Exercise: `4`
- Reps: 2-3
- Sets: 2-3

☑ **TOE RAISE/CALF RAISE**
- Exercise: `7`
- Reps: 8-10
- Sets: 2-3

☑ **LUNGES**
- Exercise: `14`
- Reps: 8-10
- Sets: 2-3

☑ **TORSO STRETCH**
- Exercise: `29`
- Reps: 8-10
- Sets: 2-3

☑ **BRIDGES**
- Exercise: `34`
- Reps: 8-10
- Sets: 2-3

☑ **FULL BODY STRETCH #2**
- Exercise: `37`
- Reps: 5-6
- Sets: 1-3

☑ **FOREARM STRETCH**
- Exercise: `57`
- Reps: hold for 10-30 seconds
- Sets: 1

☑ **SHOULDER DOORWAY STRETCH #1**
- Exercise: `43`
- Reps: 1-3
- Sets: 2-3

PROGRAM: WEEK #2

☑ **ANKLE INVERSION**
- Exercise: `5`
- Reps: 5-10
- Sets: 1

☑ **ANKLE EVERSION**
- Exercise: `6`
- Reps: 5-10
- Sets: 1

☑ **STAIRSTEP HAMSTRING RAISE**
- Exercise: `12`
- Reps: hold for 10-30 seconds
- Sets: 2-3

☑ **TORSO ROTATION**
- Exercise: `30`
- Reps: 8-10
- Sets: 2-3

☑ **TRUNK LIFTS**
- Exercise: `28`
- Reps: 4-5
- Sets: 2-3

☑ **ARM CIRCLES**
- Exercise: `47`
- Reps: 10-12
- Sets: 1

☑ **FINGER STRETCH**
- Exercise: `59`
- Reps: 5-6
- Sets: 1

☑ **WRIST/FOREARM STRETCH**
- Exercise: `60`
- Reps: 2-3
- Sets: 1

PROGRAM: WEEK #3

- ☑ **STAIRSTEP CALF RAISE**
  - Exercise: `8`
  - Reps: 5-6
  - Sets: 2-3

- ☑ **HAMSTRING DOORWAY STRETCH**
  - Exercise: `13`
  - Reps: hold for 20-30 seconds
  - Sets: 2-3

- ☑ **LOWER TRUNK ROTATION**
  - Exercise: `39`
  - Reps: 8-10
  - Sets: 2-3

- ☑ **STANDING TWISTS**
  - Exercise: `40`
  - Reps: 8-10
  - Sets: 2-3

- ☑ **FULL BODY STRETCH #1**
  - Exercise: `36`
  - Reps: 5-6
  - Sets: 2-3

- ☑ **ROTATOR CUFF TOWEL PULL**
  - Exercise: `56`
  - Reps: 1-2
  - Sets: 2

- ☑ **CAT CURL**
  - Exercise: `64`
  - Reps: 5-10
  - Sets: 2-3

- ☑ **COW CURL**
  - Exercise: `63`
  - Reps: 5-10
  - Sets: 2-3

PROGRAM: WEEK #4

- ☑ **SIDE-LYING QUAD STRETCH**
  - Exercise: `15`
  - Reps: 2-3
  - Sets: 2-3

- ☑ **HAMSTRING WITH TOWEL**
  - Exercise: `21`
  - Reps: hold for 10-30 seconds
  - Sets: 2-3

- ☑ **RESISTANCE BAND CLAMSHELLS**
  - Exercise: `22`
  - Reps: hold for 1-2 seconds
  - Sets: 2-3

- ☑ **BACK EXTENSION #2**
  - Exercise: `26`
  - Reps: 5-6
  - Sets: 2-3

- ☑ **KNEES TO CHEST**
  - Exercise: `33`
  - Reps: 2-3
  - Sets: 2-3

- ☑ **SEATED TWISTS**
  - Exercise: `38`
  - Reps: 8-10
  - Sets: 2-3

- ☑ **TRICEPS PUSH**
  - Exercise: `58`
  - Reps: hold for 5-10 seconds
  - Sets: 1-2

- ☑ **SNOW ANGELS**
  - Exercise: `62`
  - Reps: 15-20
  - Sets: 1

PROGRAM: WEEK #5

☑ **PRONE QUAD**
- Exercise: **16**
- Reps: 2-3
- Sets: 1

☑ **STABILITY BALL WALL SQUATS**
- Exercise: **23**
- Reps: 3-5
- Sets: 2-3

☑ **SEATED GROIN STRETCH**
- Exercise: **18**
- Reps: 8-10
- Sets: 2-3

☑ **BACK EXTENSION #2**
- Exercise: **26**
- Reps: 5-6
- Sets: 2-3

☑ **STANDING TWISTS**
- Exercise: **40**
- Reps: 8-10
- Sets: 2-3

☑ **SHOULDER DOORWAY STRETCH #2**
- Exercise: **44**
- Reps: hold for 20-30 seconds
- Sets: 1-2

☑ **WALL WALK**
- Exercise: **53**
- Reps: hold for 10 seconds
- Sets: 2-3

☑ **FOREARM STRETCH**
- Exercise: **57**
- Reps: hold for 10-30 seconds
- Sets: 1

PROGRAM: WEEK #6

☑ **LEG EXTENSIONS**
- Exercise: **10**
- Reps: 8-10
- Sets: 2-3

☑ **TOE RAISE/CALF RAISE**
- Exercise: **7**
- Reps: hold for 10 seconds
- Sets: 2-3

☑ **BACK EXTENSION #3**
- Exercise: **27**
- Reps: 8-10
- Sets: 2-3

☑ **STANDING SIDE BENDS**
- Exercise: **31**
- Reps: 8-10
- Sets: 2-3

☑ **SEATED TWISTS**
- Exercise: **38**
- Reps: 8-10
- Sets: 2-3

☑ **CHIN TUCK**
- Exercise: **50**
- Reps: 3-5
- Sets: 2

☑ **HEAD TURN**
- Exercise: **48**
- Reps: 3-5
- Sets: 2

☑ **NECK TILT**
- Exercise: **49**
- Reps: 3-5
- Sets: 2

PROGRAM: WEEK #7

☑ **FOOT/ANKLE CIRCLES**
- Exercise: `3`
- Reps: 10-20
- Sets: 1

☑ **HAMSTRING LEAN FORWARD**
- Exercise: `11`
- Reps: 8-10
- Sets: 2-3

☑ **ACHILLES WALL STRETCH**
- Exercise: `24`
- Reps: hold for 20-30 seconds
- Sets: 2-3

☑ **FULL BODY STRETCH #1**
- Exercise: `36`
- Reps: 8-10
- Sets: 2-3

☑ **BRIDGES**
- Exercise: `34`
- Reps: 8-10
- Sets: 2-3

☑ **TORSO ROTATION**
- Exercise: `30`
- Reps: 8-10
- Sets: 2-3

☑ **SHOULDER SQUEEZE**
- Exercise: `45`
- Reps: 2-3
- Sets: 2-3

☑ **ARM SWINGS**
- Exercise: `52`
- Reps: 10-20
- Sets: 1

PROGRAM: WEEK #8

☑ **TOE RAISE/CALF RAISE**
- Exercise: `7`
- Reps: hold for 10 seconds
- Sets: 1-2

☑ **LEG SWINGS**
- Exercise: `19`
- Reps: 10-20
- Sets: 1-2

☑ **MODIFIED SQUATS**
- Exercise: `20`
- Reps: 4-5
- Sets: 2-3

☑ **TORSO STRETCH**
- Exercise: `29`
- Reps: 8-10
- Sets: 2-3

☑ **LOWER TRUNK ROTATION**
- Exercise: `39`
- Reps: 8-10
- Sets: 2-3

☑ **SHOULDER ROLL**
- Exercise: `46`
- Reps: 5-10
- Sets: 2-3

☑ **PENDULUM**
- Exercise: `51`
- Reps: 10-20
- Sets: 1

☑ **ROTATOR CUFF ELBOW PULL #1**
- Exercise: `54`
- Reps: 8-10
- Sets: 2-3

ACE inhibitor: A drug used to treat high blood pressure by reducing the resistance of arteries.

Alzheimer's disease: A progressive, degenerative disorder that attacks nerve cells in the brain and causes loss of memory, thinking and language skills, and behavioral changes.

antidepressants: Drugs used to treat clinically diagnosed depression and other conditions.

antihypertensives: Drugs used to reduce high blood pressure.

arthroplasty: Surgical repair or replacement of a joint.

autoimmune: An overactive immune response in which the body attacks its own tissues and cells.

balance: The even distribution of weight that enables a person to remain upright and steady; also called equilibrium.

benign paroxysmal positional vertigo: A brief sensation of dizziness, confusion, or disorientation.

beta-blockers: Drugs that interfere with the ability of adrenaline to stimulate the beta receptors of the heart.

body mass index: A formula for categorizing weight in relation to height.

cataracts: Cloudiness of the eye's lens.

cognitive processing speed: How quickly a person can perform relatively easy cognitive tasks.

dementia: A loss of mental ability that interferes with normal daily activities.

diabetic retinopathy: A condition in which diabetes has affected the eyes by damaging the blood vessels of the retina.

diuretic: A drug that causes an increase in the excretion of urine.

electromyogram: A record of the electrical activity of a muscle.

flexibility: The range of motion through which a joint moves.

gait training: An activity that trains or retrains a person to walk, usually after a stroke or other traumatic event.

geriatrician: A physician who specializes in the treatment of older people.

glaucoma: Loss of sight caused by increased pressure within the eyeball.

glitazones: A class of medicines that may be used for the treatment of type 2 diabetes.

HDL: High density lipoprotein; a type of lipoprotein that removes cholesterol deposits from the arteries and protects against coronary disease.

hyponatremia: Decreased levels of sodium in the blood.

labyrinthitis: An infection or inflammation of the inner ear.

macular degeneration: A disease in which the cells of the macula degenerate, resulting in blurred vision.

Meniere's disease: A disorder of the inner ear that causes vertigo.

metabolic syndrome: A group of symptoms that increase the risk of heart disease and other health problems.

mobility: The ability to move in one's environment with ease and without restriction.

multiple sclerosis: A disease in which the protective myelin sheath that covers nerves slowly deteriorates.

narcotics: Also called opioids, may be prescribed for severe pain, and are highly addictive.

obesity: A higher level of being overweight in relation to height, sometimes defined as being 20 percent or more over healthy weight.

orthostatic hypotension: Low blood pressure that occurs immediately when a person stands up after a period of sitting or lying down; also called postural hypotension.

osteoarthritis (OA): A disease characterized by the degeneration of cartilage and the underlying bone.

osteopenia: Lower-than-normal bone density.

osteoporosis: A disease in which the bones become weak, brittle, and porous.

otolaryngologist: A physician who specializes in conditions of the ear, nose, and throat.

overpronation: A movement of the foot in which it rolls excessively inward when the person takes a step or runs.

overweight: A weight that is not healthy for a person of a given height.

Parkinson's disease: A condition that results from the loss of brain cells that produce dopamine, a hormone that affects movement.

perilymph fistula: A condition in which the fluid of the inner ear leaks to the middle ear.

peripheral neuropathy: A condition associated with diabetes in which the peripheral nerves are damaged.

polypharmacy: Taking several medications (usually five or more) to treat a condition or conditions.

PNF stretching: Proprioceptive neuromuscular facilitation, a technique most often used in clinical or rehabilitation settings that combines stretching, isometric contractions, relaxing a muscle, and restretching it.

postural sway: The body sway that results from messages received by nerves in the ear that help a person maintain balance.

pronation: The way the foot and ankle move after the foot strikes the ground.

proprioception: Awareness of the position and movement of the body.

quad cane: A walking cane with four small supports that contact the floor.

resistance training: A form of exercise that involves movement or attempted movement against resistance (or load).

rheumatoid arthritis (RA): The most debilitating type of arthritis and an inflammatory disease thought to cause the body's immune system to attack the lining of the joints.

rotator cuff: A group of muscles that surround the shoulder joint.

sarcopenia: Age-related loss of muscle mass and strength.

sedatives: Drugs that soothe or calm a person, ease agitation, and permit sleep.

stroke: A condition that occurs when the flow of blood to the brain is interrupted, causing the sudden death of brain cells.

supination: The action of the feet in which they roll outward when running or walking; also called underpronation.

vestibular neuronitis: An infection, usually a virus, of the vestibular nerve.

vertigo: A sensation of dizziness.

American Academy Of Orthopaedic Surgeons
www.aaos.org
847-823-7186
9400 West Higgins Rd.
Rosemont, IL 60018

American Academy Of Physical Medicine & Rehabilitation
www.aapmr.org
847-227-6000
9700 West Bryn Mawr Ave.
Suite 200
Rosemont, IL 60018-5701

American College Of Sports Medicine
www.acsm.org
317-637-9200
401 West Michigan St.
Indianapolis, IN 46202-3233

American Council On Exercise
www.acefitness.org
888-825-3636
4851 Paramount Dr.
San Diego, CA 92123

American Heart Association
www.heart.org
800-242-8721
7272 Greenville Ave.
Dallas, TX 75231

American Orthopaedic Foot & Ankle Society
www.aofas.org
800-235-4855
9400 West Higgins Rd.
Suite 220
Rosemont, IL 60018

American Physical Therapy Association
www.apta.org
800-999-2782
3030 Potomac Ave.
Suite 100
Alexandria, VA 22305-3085

American Podiatric Medical Association
www.apma.org
301-581-9200
9312 Old Georgetown Rd.
Bethesda, MD 20814-1621

Arthritis Foundation
www.arthritis.org
404-872-7100
1355 Peachtree St., NE
Suite 600
Atlanta, GA 30309

Centers For Disease Control & Prevention
www.cdc.gov
800-232-4636
1600 Clifton Rd.
Atlanta, GA 30329-4027

Center For Healthy Aging
www.ncoa.org
202-479-1200
c/o National Council on Aging
251 18th St., S.
Suite 500
Arlington, VA 22202

Department Of Rehabilitation Services
www.rehab.ucla.edu
310-825-5650
UCLA Health System
757 Westwood Blvd.
Suite 3127
Los Angeles, CA 90094

National Association For Health And Fitness
https://www.physicalfitness.org/
518-456-1058
10 Kings Mill Ct.
Albany, NY 12205-3632

National Council On Aging
www.ncoa.org
571-527-3900
251 18th St., S
Suite 500
Arlington, VA 22202

National Institute On Aging
www.nia.nih.gov
800-222-2225
31 Center Dr.
MSC 2292
Bethesda, MD 20892

National Safety Council
www.nsc.org
800-621-7615
1121 Spring Lake Dr.
Itasca, IL 60143-3201

National Strength & Conditioning Association
www.nsca.com
719-632-6722
1885 Bob Johnson Dr.
Colorado Springs, CO 80906

Office Of Disease Prevention And Health Promotion
www.health.gov
email: odphpinfo@hhs.gov
U.S. Department of Health and Human Services
Tower Bldg.
1101 Wootton Pkwy.
Suite LL100
Rockville, MD 20852

President's Council On Fitness, Sports & Nutrition
www.fitness.gov
240-276-9567
1101 Wootton Pkwy.
Suite 560
Rockville, MD 20852

U.S. Department Of Veterans Affairs
www.move.va.gov
www.patientsafety.va.gov
810 Vermont Ave., NW
Washington, DC 20420

YMCA Of The USA
www.ymca.net
800-872-9622
101 North Wacker Dr.
Suite 1600
Chicago, IL 60606

Not sure how often to walk or for how long? No problem. Use this walking program as your guide and then adapt it to your needs. Remember to also do flexibility and strengthening activities each week and to warm up and cool down by walking slowly for 5 minutes before and after walking briskly.

		PACE	TIME EACH DAY	NUMBER OF DAYS	TOTAL TIME FOR THE WEEK
Month 1	Week 1	Slow	10 minutes	4 days	40 min
	Week 2	Slow	10 minutes	4 days	40 min
	Week 3	Slow	15 minutes	5 days	1 hr 15 min
	Week 4	Slow – Brisk	20 minutes	5 days	1 hr 40 min
Month 2	Week 5	Brisk	30 minutes	5 days	2 hrs 30 min
	Week 6	Brisk	25 minutes	6 days	2 hrs 30 min
	Week 7	Brisk	30 minutes	5 days	2 hrs 30 min
	Week 8	Brisk	35 minutes	5 days	2 hrs 55 min

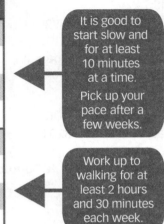

It is good to start slow and for at least 10 minutes at a time.

Pick up your pace after a few weeks.

Work up to walking for at least 2 hours and 30 minutes each week.

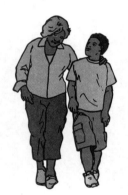

Need some help getting started? Try these tips:

• Walk with a friend. You can motivate each other to do it each week.

• Walk when you have a break in your day. This might be during lunch, after dropping the kids off at school, or at the end of your work day.

• Track your time and progress to help stay on course.

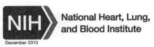
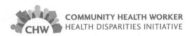
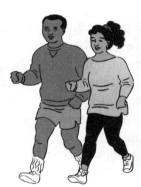

National Heart, Lung, and Blood Institute

December 2013

COMMUNITY HEALTH WORKER
HEALTH DISPARITIES INITIATIVE